TRAINING MANUAL FOR
INTRAVENOUS ADMIXTURE PERSONNEL,
FIFTH EDITION

by

Max L. Hunt Jr., M.S., R.Ph.
Director, Department of Pharmacy
University of Kentucky Hospital
Lexington, Kentucky

Edited by

Vicente J. Tormo, M.S., R.Ph.
Senior Pharmacy Consultant
Baxter Healthcare Corporation
Round Lake, Illinois

This title is co-published with Precept Press. For quantity discounts and order information, call: Precept Press, 1-800-225-3775 (outside Illinois); 312-467-0424.

8
RM170
, H85 x

CONTENTS

PREFACE

As pharmacy practice moves to a more patient-centered concept of pharmaceutical care, pharmacists will rely more than ever on new and expanded roles for support personnel. Technicians will assume many of the traditional drug distribution responsibilities to free pharmacists to provide direct patient care. Quality training programs are needed to prepare support personnel to assume these new and expanded roles. Some training programs for pharmacy support personnel are quite extensive and achieve excellent results. More often, however, programs are simply-on-the-job training that lack sufficient planning for maximum accomplishment in a minimum amount of time.

The purpose of this training manual is to provide a basis for conducting a well-organized training program for pharmacy personnel involved in preparing intravenous admixtures. The manual allows trainees to learn at their own speed, provides material for review throughout the training period, and serves as a reference after the training program is completed. Although this manual is intended primarily for training I.V. admixture technicians, the material may also be useful for training pharmacy students, as well as pharmacists or other health care providers who have had little or no previous training in this area.

This manual assumes no prior knowledge of drugs, equipment, or techniques on the part of the trainee; the only prerequisite is a basic understanding of mathematics. The manual has been made as complete as was practical, recognizing that detailed techniques may differ, depending upon the I.V. administration system used and the policies and procedures of a specific pharmacy department. The techniques described in this manual are recommended procedures and do not necessarily represent the only acceptable methods in use.

It is suggested that a coordinated training program be designed to integrate this training manual with the pharmacy department's policy and procedure manual. These two resources can serve as the basis for any classroom instruction. An equally important component is the practical training a technician must receive in order to progressively participate in each phase of processing admixture orders. The practical portion of the training should be coordinated with the classroom instruction so that each reinforces the other to facilitate more effective learning. The practical training should allow the training to perform those tasks that have been taught as soon as possible in order to gain experience and confidence, to provide a base upon which further instruction can be built, and to allow the trainee a feeling of participation and contribution.

CHAPTER 1

INTRODUCTION TO THE INTRAVENOUS ADMIXTURE PROGRAM

Intravenous solutions are commonly administered to patients who are cared for in hospitals, long-term care facilities, home care programs, infusion centers, and emergency transport vehicles such as ambulances and helicopters. They are used extensively to replace body fluids and to serve as a vehicle for injecting drugs into the body. Special education and training are required by personnel who prepare and administer sterile intravenous solutions, frequently referred to simply as *I.V. solutions.*

One or more drugs are commonly added to the I.V. solution to prepare the final sterile product. The drug is referred to as the *additive* and the final product is referred to as the *admixture*.

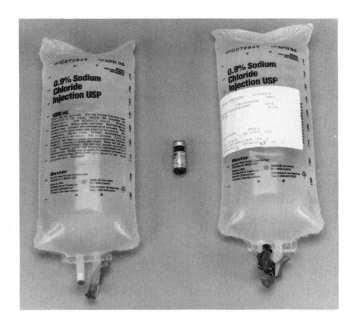

FIGURE 1.1. COMPONENTS OF AN I.V. ADMIXTURE

RESPONSIBILITY FOR PREPARING ADMIXTURES

Because the compounding of I.V. admixtures clearly is drug preparation, it is appropriately the responsibility of a pharmacist. Support for this point of view can be found in standards published by the Joint Commission on Accreditation of Healthcare Organizations (JCAHO), by the American Society of Health-System Pharmacists (ASHP), and by the National Coordinating Committee on Large Volume Parenterals (NCCLVP). JCAHO is a national organization that establishes standards of practice for various health care organizations and is the agency responsible for accrediting hospitals in the United States. ASHP is the national professional organization for pharmacists practicing in health system organizations. NCCLVP is an interdisciplinary group of health professionals gathered to review methods of compounding intravenous admixtures.

JCAHO standards are undergoing significant modification as they focus on functions and processes (e.g., assessment of patients; treatment of patients) rather than individual departments. Although previous JCAHO standards have specifically required pharmacy preparation of I.V. admixtures in all but emergency situations, beginning in 1994 they have become less prescriptive as to who performs a task as long as it is done appropriately. JCAHO's *1995 Comprehensive Accreditation Manual for Hospitals*, (JCAHO, Oakbrook Terrace, IL, 1994) states, in part:

Section 1: Care of Patients, Medication Use
TX.3   The organization has a functioning mechanism designed to ensure the safe use of medication. The design of this mechanism is based on a framework that addresses the following:

TX.3.2   The preparation and dispensing of medication(s) including

3.2.1   adherence to applicable law, regulation, licensure, and professional standards of practice;

3.2.2   appropriate control of medications;

3.2.3   a patient medication dose system;

3.2.4   the review of prescriptions or orders by a pharmacist

Intent of TX.3.2.2 through TX.3.2.4
The organization develops and maintains a mechanism designed to ensure the safe and accurate dispensing of medications. The mechanism includes a review of each prescription or order for medication, with input from the prescriber or orderer if questions arise. The mechanism also addresses a standard method for appropriately and safely labeling medications dispensed to both inpatients and outpatients. In addition, medications are dispensed in as ready-to-administer forms as possible to minimize the need for further manipulations that introduce opportunities for error. ...

Because this standard is now less detailed and prescriptive, pharmacy practice standards, such as those published by the ASHP, must be consulted for contemporary interpretation.

ASHP's document, *ASHP Guidelines: Minimum Standards for Pharmacies in Institutions* (Am J Hosp Pharm 1985;42:372-5), states, in part:

Standard III: Drug Distribution and Control

• • •

Pharmacy personnel shall prepare all sterile products (e.g., chemotherapy injections, continuous and intermittent I.V. preparations, irrigation solutions), except in emergencies.

Another document, *ASHP Technical Assistance Bulletin on Hospital Drug Distribution and Control* (Am J Hosp Pharm 1980;37:1097-1103), states, in part:

The Medication System...Medication Distribution

• • •

(8) Intravenous Admixture Services. The preparation of sterile products (e.g., I.V. admixtures, "piggy-backs," irrigations) is an important part of the drug control system. The pharmacy is responsible for assuring that all

such products used in the institution are: (1) therapeutically and pharmaceutically appropriate (i.e., are rational and free of incompatibilitiies or similar problems) for the patient; (2) free from microbial and pyrogenic contaminants; (3) free from unacceptable levels of particulate and other toxic contaminants; (4) correctly prepared (i.e., contain the correct amounts of the correct drugs), and (5) properly labeled, stored, and distributed. Centralizing all sterile compounding procedures within the pharmacy department is the best way to achieve these goals.

Additionally, the National Coordinating Committee on Large Volume Parenterals adopted a statement (Recommended methods for compounding intravenous admixtures in hospitals. Am J Hosp Pharm 1975;32:261-70), which states, in part:

Section II D, Compounding Responsibilities

1. The compounding of LVPs (large volume parenterals) is a professional function requiring the expertise of a licensed pharmacist in all but emergency situations when a pharmacist is unavailable.

2. LVPs can usually be best prepared in a centrally located pharmacy.

• • •

There are certain advantages to having a pharmacy admixture program. A pharmacy I.V. admixture program:

1. Centralizes the responsibility for compounding, dispensing, and controlling parenteral admixtures.
2. Reduces the need for nurses and physicians to compound admixtures, providing them additional time for their professional responsibilities.
3. Standardizes the labeling of admixture solutions.
4. Provides effective control over the use of unstable, deteriorated, or outdated drugs in admixtures.
5. Provides for proper screening of incompatibilities in drug admixtures.
6. Provides the proper controlled environmental conditions during the compounding process through the use of a laminar air flow hood.
7. Provides accuracy in the calculation of the quantity of components and the compounding process.
8. Makes possible individualized tailoring of solutions and additives to meet the specific needs of the patient.

TECHNICIAN RESPONSIBILITIES

A technician is a person skilled in a specific technical process or type of work. Many health care professions—most notably medicine, dentistry, and nursing—use supportive personnel to perform duties formerly done only by professionally trained and licensed personnel. A pharmacy technician who compounds I.V. admixtures under the direct supervision of a pharmacist is an example of how support personnel in health care organizations are assuming increasingly important roles. Several factors are contributing to an expanded role for pharmacy technicians:

1. The profession of pharmacy is moving toward the philosophy of *pharmaceutical care*, which is the direct, responsible provision of medication-related care for the purpose of achieving definite outcomes that improve a patient's quality of life. As the pharmacist becomes more involved in providing direct patient care, support personnel will assume many of the drug distribution responsibilities done by pharmacists.

2. A national movement supported by many pharmacy organizations favors the voluntary certification of technicians, a move that should result in more competent support personnel capable of assuming these expanded roles.
3. Many state boards of pharmacy have a more flexible attitude toward a legitimate, well-defined role for pharmacy technicians. This can be seen in the fact that several states have recognized pharmacy technicians in state board regulations and a few even permit credentialed technicians to check other technicians in limited situations.

However, in many states, the state board of pharmacy still imposes severe limitations on the activities of pharmacy technicians. Thus, technicians in some states may not be allowed to perform the procedures described in this training manual. Directors of pharmacy must investigate what limitations apply to the use of technicians in their specific situation before instituting any program using support personnel.

An I.V. admixture technician commonly performs the following duties, depending on the policies of the particular pharmacy department and the limitations imposed by the state board of pharmacy:

- Prepares complete, uniform labels
- Gathers and assembles drugs and solutions to be used in compounding each admixture
- Reconstitutes drug additives, using appropriate aseptic technique
- Compounds the admixture, using appropriate aseptic technique
- Checks the admixture for clarity and presence of particulate matter
- Labels the admixture, including the assignment of an expiration date
- Maintains a patient profile so that admixtures can be prepared and delivered to the nursing unit when needed
- Enters data, such as the admixture order, into a pharmacy computer and requests data, such as labels or profiles, from the computer system
- Delivers completed admixtures to the patient care area and returns unused admixtures to the pharmacy
- Restocks the admixture area
- Maintains work load records
- Initiates patient charges for admixtures administered and credits for admixtures returned unused
- Maintains the admixture area in a neat and orderly manner

PHARMACIST RESPONSIBILITIES

A pharmacist working with a pharmacy technician is responsible for coordinating the preparation of admixtures and for supervising all activities of the technician. Responsibilities of this individual include the following duties:

- Interprets physicians' orders, consulting with nursing and medical staff members when necessary. Every new admixture prescription received in the pharmacy must be checked by a registered pharmacist, inasmuch as the pharmacist has legal responsibility for the accuracy of medications dispensed from the pharmacy. Thus, a pharmacist must interpret the prescription for accuracy, dosage, rate of administration, compatibility, stability, and mathematical calculations needed.

- Oversees the proper storage and handling of drugs in the I.V. admixture area
- Assures that proper labeling practices are followed
- Assures that technicians follow proper aseptic technique in preparing I.V. admixtures
- Checks the patient profile or computer entry against the original prescription order for accuracy
- Checks the completed I.V. admixture for accuracy and clarity. Having assumed ultimate responsibility for accurate preparation, only a pharmacist should perform the final check of the end product. Documentation must include identification (e.g., initials) of the responsible pharmacist.
- Coordinates the overall needs of the nursing and medical staffs for essential pharmaceutical services (e.g., delivery schedules, emergency admixtures, specially prepared admixtures, etc.)

PERSONAL ATTITUDE

In compounding and dispensing medications, the pharmacist's primary concerns must be safety, accuracy, and appropriateness. Both pharmacists and technicians must adhere to high standards of performance and conduct in order to provide accurate, high-quality admixture products and service.

A responsible, conscientious attitude is extremely important when preparing I.V. admixtures. Mistakes that could be harmful to the patient could easily go unnoticed unless both the pharmacist and the technician have the right attitude to guide their conduct. For example, if a pharmacist or technician suspects that he or she may have accidentally contaminated an I.V. admixture, either would be obligated to discard that admixture and start over. Likewise, pharmacy managers must willingly support, rather than reprimand, a pharmacist or technician for admitting to a possible break in technique, even though it results in wasted product. In the interest of good patient care, it is imperative that all personnel involved in the preparation of I.V. admixtures display a responsible, conscientious attitude toward the important work they perform.

CHAPTER 2

INTRAVENOUS ADMINISTRATION

MEDICATION ADMINISTRATION

Medications may be administered in numerous ways, depending on the dosage form, characteristics of a particular drug, and the specific needs of the patient. Many, but not all, medications are available in several dosage forms. For example, ampicillin is available as a capsule, oral suspension, and injection. Other drugs may be available as tablets, oral solutions, ointments, etc. Some drugs have an injectable form, but not an oral form—and vice-versa.

Medications intended for injection can be administered by several different routes. The most common injectable routes of administration are *intravenous*, *intramuscular*, and *subcutaneous* (just under the skin). Although most products prepared in an I.V. admixture area of the pharmacy are intended for intravenous use, other products commonly prepared might include dialysis solutions, *cardioplegia solutions* (solutions used in heart surgery), irrigation solutions, or epidural infusions.

Regardless of how a medication is administered, it is not beneficial until it reaches the blood and is distributed throughout the body. A medication that is administered orally must be absorbed across the wall of the digestive tract to reach the blood circulation. Likewise, drugs injected intramuscularly must be absorbed through tissue membranes and into the bloodstream. Often, some of the drug administered by these routes does not cross these barriers efficiently, so the amount of drug reaching the blood is somewhat less than the amount administered.

ADVANTAGES AND DISADVANTAGES OF INTRAVENOUS ADMINISTRATION

Intravenous administration of medication (figure 2.1) has certain advantages over other routes:

1. I.V. administration provides the most rapid onset of action.
2. The medication is administered directly into the blood stream so that absorption across a barrier is not necessary.
3. Patients may not be able to take medication by mouth because they are unconscious, uncooperative, nauseated, or vomiting.
4. A particular medication may not be suitable or available for oral administration. For example, insulin cannot be given by mouth because it is destroyed in the stomach. Other drugs are not destroyed, but are simply not absorbed when administered orally.

Certain dangers and disadvantages are also associated with medications administered intravenously:

1. The effects of an error in a dose are magnified when a medication is given intravenously because it is rapidly distributed upon injection. Once administered, it is difficult to stop the drug from producing all of its effects, including adverse effects.
2. A risk of infection is always present whenever the skin is punctured.
3. Pain, real or psychological, may accompany an injection. Some medications are irritating when injected and may cause local tissue damage or soreness.
4. Medications injected intravenously must be sterile. This demands special drug dosage forms and supplies, as well as skills to prepare and administer these drugs.

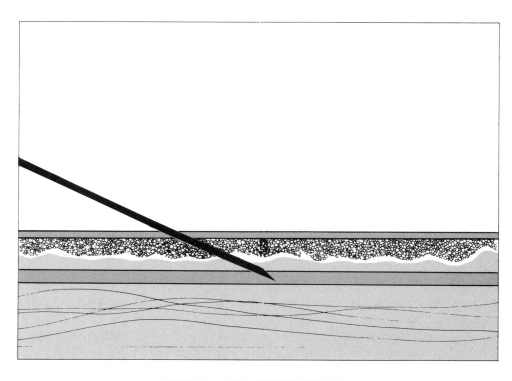

FIGURE 2.1. INTRAVENOUS INJECTION

OTHER RATIONALE FAVORING THE INTRAVENOUS ROUTE

Intravenous administration, made directly into a vein, is a very predictable route of parenteral administration. The dose is precisely known because the drug bypasses all barriers to absorption. Onset of drug action by this route is rapid because it is distributed throughout the body in only a few minutes.

Medications that are too irritating to be given by one of the other injectable routes may possibly be given intravenously provided the rate of administration is slow. The inner lining of the vein is relatively insensitive to pain, and the drug is further diluted by the large volume of blood. With the other injectable routes (e.g., intramuscular), the medication remains undiluted in a relatively confined area. Dilution of a drug before I.V. administration also helps reduce irritation. Such dilution for other injectable routes of administration is limited because tissue can accommodate only a small volume of fluid.

Only medications in aqueous solutions should be introduced intravenously. Suspensions of drugs or drugs in oil generally are not administered intravenously, although there are exceptions, such as I.V. fat emulsions.

Several differences between arteries and veins may explain why veins are preferred to arteries for the administration of drugs and solutions:

1. Veins can expand when a large volume of fluid is introduced.
2. Veins are located closer to the surface of the skin and are therefore more readily accessible for injection.

3. Pressure inside a vein (*back pressure*) is relatively low compared to that in an artery and can be overcome by an I.V. solution allowed to flow freely into the vein by gravity alone. However, because the back pressure inside an artery may be 6 to 10 times greater than that in a vein, special techniques or equipment are needed to force the drug into the artery.

TYPES OF INTRAVENOUS ADMINISTRATION

An *I.V. injection* is the administration of a relatively small volume of solution directly from a syringe. When administered over a short period, it is sometimes called an *I.V. push*. Before the medication is administered, a small volume of blood is usually drawn into the syringe (*aspirated*) to make certain that the needle is in the vein. Frequently, I.V. injections and I.V. pushes are done into an existing I.V. line or I.V. access device.

The introduction of larger volumes of solution directly into a vein is known as an *I.V. infusion*, in which the solution is permitted to flow into the vein over a relatively long period. Infusions are given to overcome dehydration, to restore depleted blood volume, and to serve as a vehicle for the administration of medications.

Infusions may be administered continuously or intermittently. *Continuous infusions* are used to administer a large volume of solution over several hours at a slow, constant rate. An example of a continuous infusion is the administration of 40 milliequivalents (mEq) of potassium chloride in 1,000 milliliters (mL or ml) of 5% dextrose injection over eight hours. *Intermittent infusions* are used to administer a relatively small volume over a short time at specific intervals. An example of an intermittent infusion is the administration of 1 g of ampicillin in 50 mL of 0.9% sodium chloride injection over 15-20 minutes every six hours.

SETUP FOR CONTINUOUS INTRAVENOUS INFUSION

Administration of an I.V. infusion requires the setup and use of special supplies and apparatus, usually consisting of the following (figure 2.2):

- A container for the solution to be administered; this is almost always a plastic bag, but may be a glass bottle
- An administration set, consisting of a spike for insertion into the solution container, a drip chamber, a length of plastic tubing, a clamp, and a needle adapter
- A needle or catheter, which is inserted into the patient's vein

The solution container is supported about three feet above the level of the injection site so that gravity causes the solution to flow from the container. A length of plastic tubing connects the solution container to the needle in the patient's vein. As the solution flows from the container, it passes through a drip chamber, which is a small reservoir connected to the plastic tubing near the solution container. By collecting in the drip chamber, the solution can flow continuously through the remainder of the tubing without mixing with air, thus avoiding the formation and administration of air bubbles. A nurse can also determine how rapidly the solution is being administered by counting the number of drops per minute that enter the drip chamber. The clamp is used to regulate the flow of the solution through the tubing. Closing the clamp progressively flattens the tubing from the "wide-open" to the "shutoff" position. At the end of the plastic tubing is a plastic needle adapter to which a needle or catheter (discussed later in this

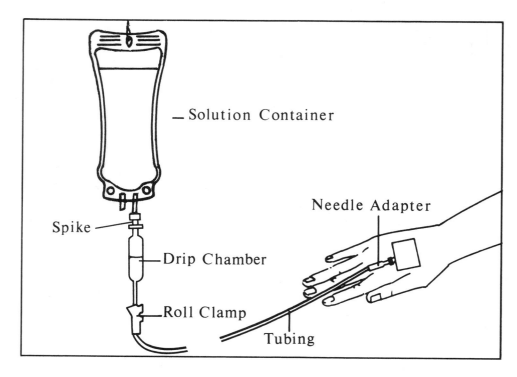

FIGURE 2.2. SETUP FOR CONTINUOUS I.V. INFUSION

chapter) is attached. All of these components are sterile and disposable in order to reduce the risk of infection. Proper technique is obviously critical to maintain that sterility.

SETUP FOR INTERMITTENT INTRAVENOUS INFUSION

Intermittent I.V. infusion involves the infusion of a medication in a relatively small volume of solution at regular intervals. During the time that the intermittent infusion is not being delivered, the large-volume continuous infusion is administered in order to keep the vein open. This setup (figure 2.3) is often referred to as a *piggyback* administration because solutions from two containers flow into the patient's vein through common tubing and a common injection site, or *venipuncture*.

One solution, generally a large-volume, continuous infusion, is sometimes designated as the *primary* solution. The other solution is usually an intermittent infusion, such as an antibiotic, that may be referred to as the *secondary*, or *piggyback* solution. The piggyback solution usually contains a medication in 50 or 100 mL of 5% dextrose injection or 0.9% sodium chloride injection. Like the primary solution container, the piggyback container is usually made of plastic and referred to as a minibag. Occasionally, the piggyback container is made of glass if the drug interacts with plastic and is referred to as a minibottle. The piggyback container may be a syringe rather than a minibag or minibottle. This is most commonly seen if the volume of solution is very small or the dose must be very precise.

The primary solution container and the piggyback solution container are connected in a "Y" type configuration shown in figure 2.3. A continuous straight administration set connects the primary solution container to the patient. This set has a "Y" injection site for the attachment of a second administration set, which is connected to the piggyback solution container. The use of these two sets together allows for the efficient, safe administration of piggyback solutions.

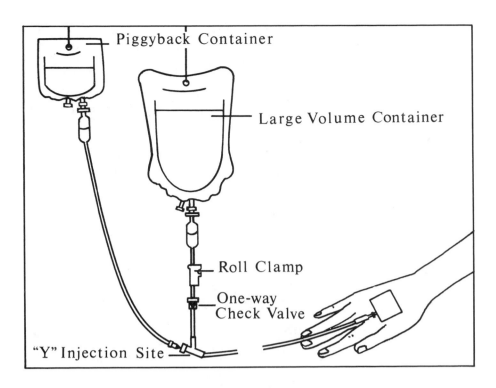

Piggyback Container

Large Volume Container

Roll Clamp

One-way
Check Valve

"Y" Injection Site

FIGURE 2.3. SETUP FOR INTERMITTENT I.V. INFUSION

First, the primary solution drip rate is established. At the appropriate time for administration of the medication, the clamp to the piggyback set can be opened to allow the piggyback solution to flow through the tubing. Because the piggyback solution is hanging higher than the primary solution, the greater pressure allows it to flow in preference to the primary solution. The piggyback solution is prevented from flowing up and into the primary solution container by a one-way check valve on the primary set. This check valve allows the solution to flow from the primary container to the patient, but not the opposite way. (Not all piggyback systems use check valves.)

Piggyback administration of medications has these advantages:

1. An additional venipuncture is not necessary.
2. Medications can be given at intervals rather than by continuous infusion, providing higher blood levels of the drug more quickly. This may lead to the more effective and rational use of many antibiotics.

The two solutions are not mixed together except within the tubing below the Y injection site. This may be important if the primary solution contains a drug that should not be combined with a drug in the secondary container because the two drugs are incompatible over a period of time.

ADMINISTRATION SETS

Administration sets have a spike insert at one end that fits into the administration set port of the solution container. The solution flows from the solution container into a drip chamber and through a length of flexible plastic tubing that has a needle adapter at the other end to which a needle or catheter is attached. Some sets have a piece of flexible rubber tubing called a Flashball device next to the needle adapter. To assure that the needle or catheter is located properly within a vein prior to starting the solution, the Flashball can be squeezed. If blood comes up into the Flashball, the needle or catheter is in the vein. A clamp on the tubing provides a means of regulating the flow rate with one hand (figure 2.4).

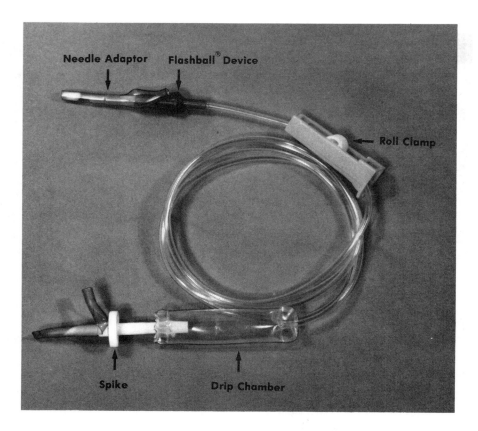

FIGURE 2.4. ADMINISTRATION SET

The typical administration set can have many variations. The spike may have an air vent built in, the drip chamber may be regular drip (e.g., 10 drops/mL) or minidrip (e.g., 60 drops/mL); the length of the tubing varies; the size of the lumen can be regular or microbore; there may or may not be a Flashball; there may be a filter incorporated into the tubing; the clamp may be a roll clamp or a slide clamp; the needle adapter may have a locking collar (Luer-Lok adapter); or there may be no drip chamber.

CATHETERS

A common alternative to inserting a needle into the patient's vein is the use of an I.V. catheter (figure 2.5). A catheter is a 1- to 5-in. piece of fine, flexible plastic tubing connected to a plastic hub. To allow insertion of a flexible catheter into the vein, the catheter has a needle inside to provide rigidity during the actual venipuncture. After insertion, the needle is pulled out, leaving the catheter in the vein. The plastic hub at the free end of the catheter is attached to a syringe or to an administration set. A catheter may be less irritating to the vein than a needle because it is more flexible; however, as with all materials foreign to the vein, inflammation increases with the length of time the catheter remains in place.

HEPARIN LOCK

A very useful device to facilitate intermittent I.V. infusions is a *heparin lock* (figure 2.6). This device attaches to an I.V. catheter or needle on one end and has a resealable rubber diaphragm at

12

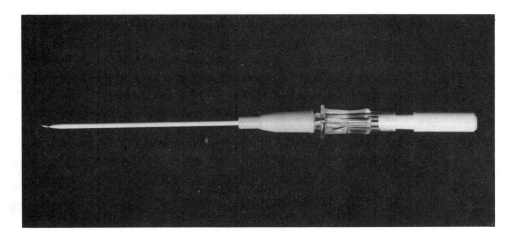

FIGURE 2.5. CATHETER

the other end. Medications can be administered intermittently through this rubber diaphragm to avoid multiple venipunctures and the need for a continuous drip primary solution to keep the vein open.

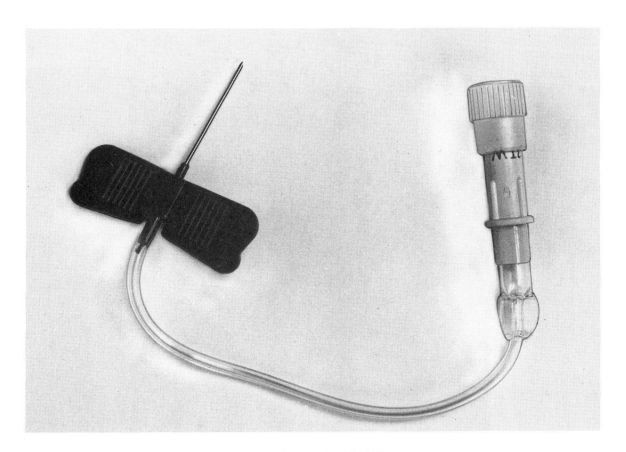

FIGURE 2.6. HEPARIN LOCK

After a drug is administered, the heparin lock is flushed with a small volume of 0.9% sodium chloride injection or a dilute heparin (an anticoagulant) solution to prevent blood clotting in the device until the next dose of medication is administered.

NEEDLELESS SYSTEMS

A recent technological advance has been the introduction of *needleless I.V. systems* to avoid the dangers of accidental needle sticks. Health care workers who draw blood from or administer parenteral medications to patients (e.g., phlebotomists, nurses) need to avoid needle sticks because exposure to a patient's blood could result in the transmission of disease such as hepatitis or AIDS. This is not a concern for individuals who work with clean needles outside of the patient care areas where they are unlikely to come in contact with blood (e.g., pharmacy personnel preparing I.V. admixtures).

The heart of the needleless system (shown below) is the injection site and the cannula. The *injection site* (figure 2.7) looks like a regular injection site used with a needle-based system, but with two basic differences: (1) the body of the injection site is somewhat larger, in order to accept the cannula

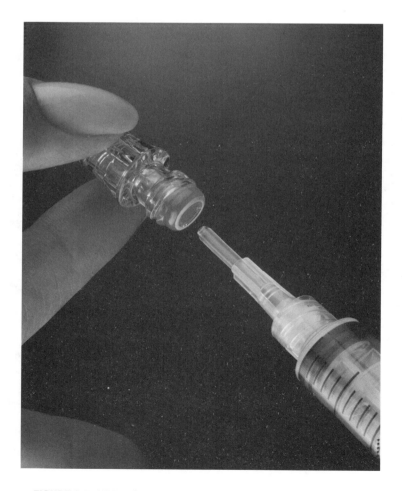

FIGURE 2.7. NEEDLELESS SYSTEM INJECTION SITE AND CANNULA

rather than a needle; and (2) the rubber cap is manufactured with a preformed slit. In some of these systems, the injection site can accept multiple cannula and needle sticks without leaking.

The plastic cannula serves the same function as a needle. However, it is shorter and broader than a needle, with a blunt tip. Thus, needle sticks are avoided. The flow rate through the cannula is equivalent to that of a 15-guage needle, one of the largest needles used in an I.V. system. The cannula can be used for delivery of parenteral solutions and for blood sampling.

To convert a regular I.V. system that uses needles to a needleless system, a needleless injection site can be inserted where a needle normally would be inserted (e.g., into the heparin lock or catheter). A cannula can be attached to the end of the administration set and then inserted into the injection site. Alternatively, a cannula can be attached to a syringe and then inserted into the injection site.

Cannulas and injection sites are available in a variety of types, e.g., with or without locking mechanisms to secure the connection between the two. Also available are administration sets that include the injection site as an integral part of the set.

The advantages of a needleless system include the following:

- Prevents accidental needle sticks and simplifies safe disposal by using cannulas rather than needles
- Helps to reduce the cost associated with needle-stick injuries
- Requires minimal change in technique, in that it is used like a conventional needle-based system

The disadvantage of a needleless system is the additional product cost.

FINAL FILTERS

Intravenous admixtures sometimes contain very small particles that may or may not be visible to the naked eye. These particles originate from the I.V. solution, the solution container, or the drug

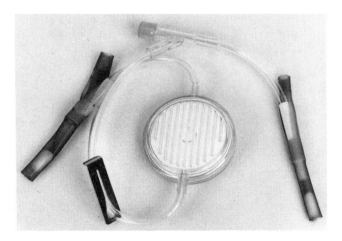

FIGURE 2.8. FINAL FILTER

additive. Particles can be harmful to some patients if they become trapped and accumulate in the small capillaries of the lungs. A filter (figure 2.8) can be used to remove these particles from I.V. admixtures as the solution is administered. A separate filter extension set can be attached to the end of the administration set so that the solution is filtered just before it enters the vein. Some administration sets incorporate a final filter as part of the set. (See chapter 8 for additional discussion on filters.)

VOLUME CONTROL CHAMBERS

A volume control chamber is a plastic cylindrical device with graduation marks along the sides to measure the volume of solution (figure 2.9). As the I.V. solution flows from the container, the device is filled to a measured volume. The clamp immediately above the volume control chamber is closed

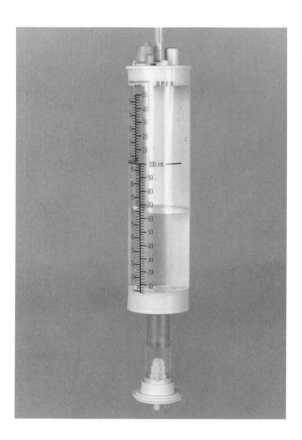

FIGURE 2.9. VOLUME CONTROL CHAMBER

when the desired volume of solution is in the unit. The volume control chamber then serves as a minicontainer from which the solution is allowed to flow when the clamp on the tubing below is opened. Medications are added to the solution through an injection port on top of the chamber. The volume control device may be a separate device, the top being inserted into the solution container and the bottom accepting the spike of the administration set. Alternatively, the volume control chamber may be an integral part of the set, located at the end of the set that is inserted into the solution container.

The volume control chamber is useful to ensure accurate measurement of the volume of fluid infused and as a safety precaution to limit the volume of fluid that may be infused accidentally.

Volume control chambers are sometimes used as piggyback containers to which medications are added, especially if the drugs are not very stable or the cumulative volume of solution from piggyback solutions presents a problem to patients who have severe fluid restrictions. Volume control sets generally are recommended only for pediatric patients, as there are normally more acceptable alternatives for other patients, as discussed previously with respect to piggyback administration.

TEMPERATURE OF THE INFUSION

When I.V. admixtures are prepared in the pharmacy, they may be compounded several hours prior to administration and stored in a refrigerator to prolong the stability period of the drug and retard bacterial growth should inadvertent contamination occur. Because a refrigerated admixture is several degrees below body temperature, there may be some concern about administering a cold solution. The admixture may be taken out of the refrigerator 20 to 30 minutes prior to administration and let stand at room temperature to warm. As the solution flows through the narrow tubing of the administration set, the large surface area exposed during that time warms the solution to near room temperature.

ADVERSE REACTIONS TO INTRAVENOUS THERAPY

The most common adverse reactions to I.V. therapy are extravasation and phlebitis. Leakage of infused medication or solution from the vein into the surrounding tissue is known as *extravasation* (or *infiltration*). Extravasation causes pain, swelling, redness, and possibly severe tissue damage if the drug is especially irritating, as are many chemotherapy drugs. Extravasation may be caused by a dislodged or misplaced catheter or needle. To minimize extravasation, blood should be aspirated into the syringe or administration set to make sure that the needle is in the vein. The patient must remain reasonably calm during the I.V. infusion to prevent dislodging the needle or catheter.

Using the same vein over a prolonged period of I.V. therapy, or administering irritating or concentrated solutions, may lead to inflammation of the vein (*phlebitis*). Symptoms include pain, burning, redness, and swelling of the immediate area.

INTRAVENOUS PUMPS AND INFUSION DEVICES

An I.V. infusion pump is a device used to control the delivery of an I.V. solution at a selected rate. A typical I.V. pump is shown in figure 2.10.

Under normal circumstances, gravity provides enough pressure to allow an I.V. solution to flow through an administration set and into the vein. The pressure generated by gravity depends on the height at which the I.V. solution is hung, but is generally sufficient to overcome the back pressure from inside the vein. However, several factors may impede the flow of solution; they include clogged filters, small (microbore) tubing or catheters, thick (viscous) solutions, and increased pressure in the vein. Pumps can be adjusted to provide just enough pressure to overcome resistance to flow and maintain a constant flow rate.

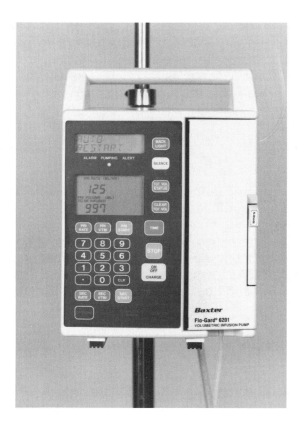

FIGURE 2.10. I.V. INFUSION PUMP

Pumps are used to:

● Assure accurate delivery of an I.V. solution, usually within 2-5% of the selected rate

● Provide an enhanced level of safety through various built-in alarms. Pumps may sound an alarm if there is air in the I.V. line or the flow of solution is impeded for any reason — for example, if a filter clogs, a patient pinches off the tubing accidentally, or the I.V. container becomes empty.

● Store data such as volume of solution already infused, infusion rate, etc.

● Save time for nurses by eliminating the need to repeatedly check on the status of the I.V. infusion

Infusion pumps are used most commonly in special care areas of a hospital, such as intensive care units and pediatric units, as well as with certain types of admixtures, such as parenteral nutrition solutions, chemotherapy solutions, and potent drugs that must be administered very accurately.

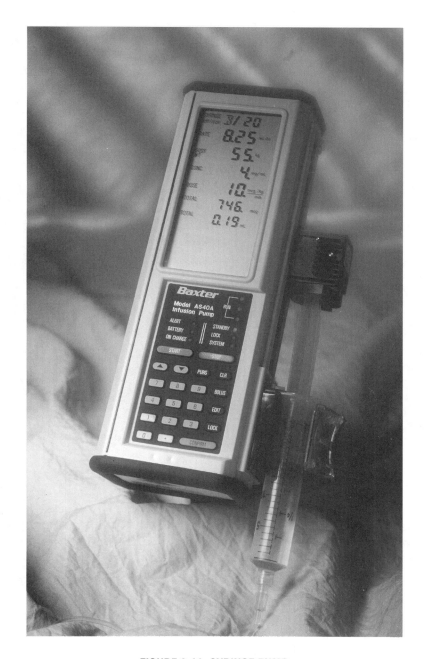

FIGURE 2.11. SYRINGE PUMP

Most I.V. pumps are designated for use in conjunction with large-volume infusions. However, many are designed to be used with a syringe to deliver the drug. Syringe pumps (figure 2.11) are most commonly used with pediatric patients, although many hospitals use syringe pumps to deliver intermittent I.V. medications as an alternative to minibags or minibottles.

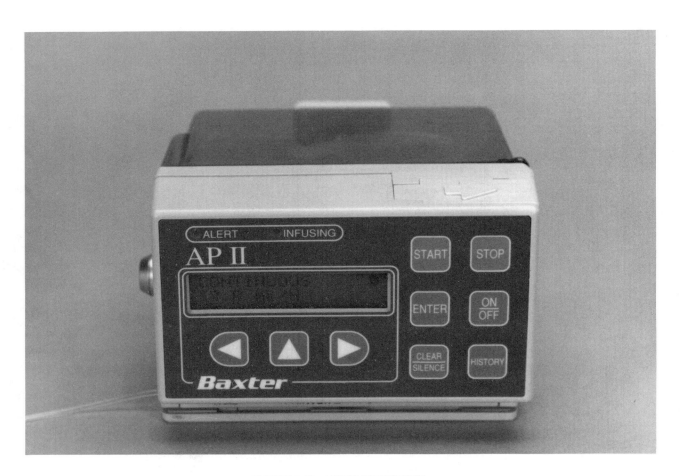

FIGURE 2.12. AMBULATORY PUMP

Smaller pumps, about the size of a hand, are also available for ambulatory patients in order to allow them greater mobility without being restrained by an infusion pump on a pole. Ambulatory pumps usually require specific tubing or drug reservoirs (e.g., bags or cassettes). An example of an ambulatory pump is shown in figure 2.12.

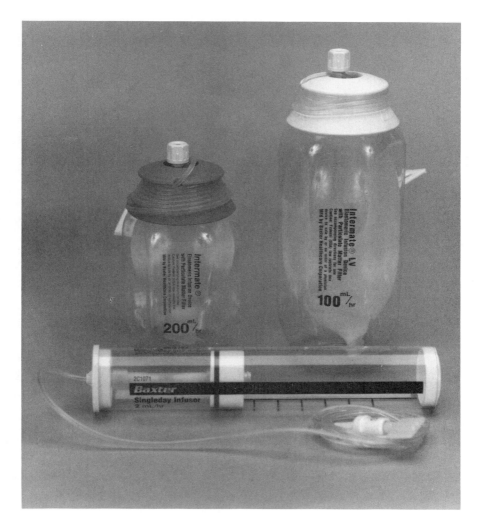

FIGURE 2.13. ELASTOMERIC INFUSION DEVICES

Another device for administering medications is the elastomeric infusion device. These devices typically consist of a balloonlike drug reservoir, encased in a hard plastic shell (figure 2.13). As the elastic reservoir contracts, it forces the medication solution out through a preattached tubing set. There is a flow restricting device in the tubing that maintains the flow of solution out of the reservoir at a constant rate. The tubing set is usually connected directly to the patient's catheter. Elastomeric infusion devices are most commonly used to deliver continuous or intermittent infusions of antibiotics, chemotherapy drugs, and pain management medications.

CHAPTER 3

INTRODUCTION TO DRUGS

Drugs are chemical compounds administered to patients in carefully regulated doses as an aid in the treatment, diagnosis, or prevention of disease. The most common use of drugs is for the treatment of disease, e.g., antibiotics to treat infection, chemotherapy drugs to treat cancer, or bronchodilators to treat asthma. Relatively few drugs are used to diagnose disease, but such uses include skin tests to diagnose allergies and radiocontrast media to visualize various organs for radiology and nuclear medicine examinations. Vaccines are a critical tool for modern societies in preventing such diseases as polio and measles; they are examples of drugs used for the prevention of disease.

Almost all drugs used in I.V. admixtures are for the treatment of disease. Antibiotics, cardio-vascular drugs, chemotherapy drugs, and electrolytes are examples of drugs used for their therapeutic effect. Vitamins and antibiotics are sometimes used prophylactically to prevent disease, and are commonly used in I.V. admixtures.

DRUG DEVELOPMENT

Most drugs are discovered through the systematic investigation of chemical compounds. Only a very small percentage of chemical compounds investigated for potential therapeutic use ever reach the market. In 1993, the average cost to bring a drug to market was about $250 million. Not only is it costly in terms of dollars, but it takes several years to take a compound from the point of discovery to a drug appearing on the market.

New drugs often are discovered by modification of existing drugs, usually through meticulous, systematic scientific screening methods. Deliberate chemical alteration of existing drugs sometimes provides drugs with significant improvements in activity or decreases in side effects. Frequently, however, this type of chemical modification makes little difference in activity.

Recently, the production of several biotechnology drugs has been made possible through advances in immunology, genetics, and molecular biology. The greatest impact has been the development of *recombinant DNA* (deoxyribonucleic acid) technology, in which very highly purified human proteins are produced in commercial quantities. Bacteria, yeast, and mammalian (e.g., mice) cells are used to replicate and "grow" proteins that the human body naturally produces in small amounts. The first recombinant DNA drug product was human insulin, approved in 1982. Current biotechnology products are used in diabetes, human growth hormone deficiency, leukemia, AIDS, heart attacks, influenza, hepatitis, dialysis anemia, and neutropenia (decreased white blood cells) caused by cancer chemotherapy. Although only about 12 biotechnology drugs have been approved so far by the U.S. Food and Drug Administration (FDA), more than 120 products are being investigated or are in the approval process. Biotechnology drugs are generally very expensive, with single doses of some drugs costing hundreds of dollars. As the recombinant DNA process is perfected, costs may be reduced. Obviously, these products must be handled carefully in the pharmacy to prevent waste.

Once a chemical substance shows promise as a drug, it is purified to its active constituents by pharmaceutical scientists. The purified substance is tested further for its pharmacological effects and then, depending on the type of drug, may be tested in laboratory animals for possible therapeutic benefits, mode of action, dosage range, and toxic reactions. If the drug shows promise in animal studies, trials are conducted to test its effectiveness and safety in humans. Patients in clinical trials of investigational drugs are volunteers. Ideally, these clinical drug trials are conducted in multiple medical centers and involve hundreds of patients to further investigate the safety and effectiveness of a new drug. The FDA is the federal agency that regulates research, production, and marketing of all drugs in the United States, both prescription and nonprescription. The FDA also conducts a postmarketing surveillance program after the drug has become available for use.

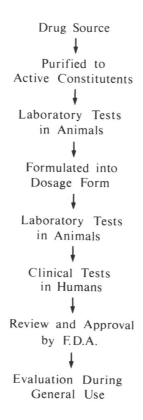

Drug Source

↓

Purified to
Active Constitutents

↓

Laboratory Tests
in Animals

↓

Formulated into
Dosage Form

↓

Laboratory Tests
in Animals

↓

Clinical Tests
in Humans

↓

Review and Approval
by F.D.A.

↓

Evaluation During
General Use

FIGURE 3.1. HOW DRUGS ARE DEVELOPED

An official drug in the United States is one that is listed in the *United States Pharmacopeia* (*USP*). The basic objectives of the *USP* are to standardize names and formulas for drugs; to provide standards and tests for the identity, purity, and quality of drugs; and to secure uniformity in biological activity. The standards assure physicians and pharmacists of dependable potency and purity for all official drugs. The initials *USP* are frequently seen following the name of a drug on official package labeling.

In hospitals and other health system organizations, a pharmacy and therapeutics committee (often referred to as the P&T committee) may impose more rigid standards for drugs used in those organizations. The committee recommends policies to the medical staff and the hospital on matters related to the therapeutic use of drugs. It is generally composed of physicians, pharmacists, and other health care professionals designated by the organization. An important function of the P & T committee is to develop and maintain a *formulary system*—an ongoing method to determine which drugs will be made available for use in the institution based upon their effectiveness, side-effect profile, and cost/ benefit. The list of accepted drugs, along with other valuable ancillary information, is published in a formulary booklet. The drugs listed are referred to as formulary drugs and are the products normally stocked by the pharmacy.

DRUG NAMES

Understanding drug names can be intimidating to individuals with no previous experience in the medical field. However, familiarity with a few principles makes the task much easier. Drugs have several names: a *chemical* name; a *generic* (*nonproprietary*) name; and a *brand* (*proprietary*) name. The table below lists typical names for drug products.

Chemical name	Generic name (nonproprietary)	Brand name (proprietary)
3, 4-dihydroxy-phenethylamine hydrochloride	dopamine	Intropin
3, 4-dihydroxy-*a*-[(isopropylamino) methyl] benzyl alcohol hydrochloride	isoproterenol	Isuprel

The chemical name of a drug is most meaningful to the pharmaceutical chemist because it describes the chemical structure of the drug; however, it is rarely used because of its complexity.

Every drug has only one generic name. Regardless of which pharmaceutical manufacturer markets the drug, it does so under the same generic name. Drugs are listed in the *USP*, most hospital formularies, textbooks, clinical studies, and noncommercial publications by their generic names.

In addition to a generic name, almost all drugs have a brand name trademarked and owned by a particular manufacturer. Although the same drug marketed by different companies has the same generic name, the brand names must be different. The brand name may appear with the sign ™ or ® at the upper right of the name to indicate that it is registered as a trademark and that its use is restricted to that company.

A drug product composed of two or more drugs is known as a *combination drug*. It has a brand name, but no single generic name. However, each component drug of the combination has a generic name. For example, Unasyn injection is a combination drug containing ampicillin and sulbactam. Most drugs used in compounding I.V. admixtures are single-entity drugs; relatively few are combination drugs.

DRUG CLASSIFICATIONS

    Drugs that have a similar effect are grouped in the same pharmacological or therapeutic classification. The following list shows the therapeutic classes of drugs frequently used in compounding I.V. admixtures. Within each therapeutic class, drugs are listed by their generic name, with the most common brand name or names of each drug shown in parentheses. (Owners of trademarks for brand names included in this list or mentioned elsewhere in this manual are given in appendix B.)

    For simplicity, generic names listed below do not include the name of their salts. For example, although *ampicillin sodium* is technically the correct generic name, *ampicillin* alone is commonly used in daily practice. Numerous references are available that list the full generic name.

1. ***Anti-infectives***
   a. Aminoglycosides

      amikacin (Amikin, Apothecon)

      gentamicin (Garamycin, Schering)

      tobramycin (Nebcin, Lilly)

   b. Cephalosporins

      cefazolin (Ancef, SmithKline Beecham; Kefzol, Lilly)

      cefotetan (Cefotan, Stuart)

      cefuroxime (Kefurox, Lilly; Zinacef, Glaxo)

      cefoxitin (Mefoxin, Merck)

        cefonicid (Monocid, SmithKline Beecham)

      cefmetazole (Zefazone, Upjohn)

      ceftizoxime (Cefizox, Fujisawa)

      cefoperazone (Cefobid, Roerig)

      ceftazidime (Fortaz, Glaxo)

        (Tazicef, SmithKline Beecham; Tazidime, Lilly)

      cefotaxime (Claforan, Hoechst-Roussel)

      ceftriaxone (Rocephin, Roche)

   c. Monobactams

      aztreonam (Azactam, Bristol-Myers Squibb)

   d. Penicillins

      mezlocillin (Mezlin, Miles)

      penicillin G (Pfizerpen, Roerig)

piperacillin (Pipracil, Lederle)

piperacillin/tazobactam (Zosyn, Lederle)

ticarcillin/clavulanic acid (Timentin, SKB)

ampicillin/sulbactam (Unasyn, Roerig)

nafcillin (Unipen, Wyeth-Ayerst)

ampicillin (Omnipen-N, Wyeth-Ayerst)

e. Tetracyclines

minocycline (Minocin, Lederle)

doxycycline (Vibramycin, Roerig)

f. Quinolones

ciprofloxacin (Cipro, Miles)

ofloxacin (Floxin, McNeil)

g. Antifungals

amphotericin B (Fungizone, Apothecon)

fluconazole (Diflucan, Roerig)

miconazole (Monistat, Janssen)

h. Miscellaneous Anti-Infectives
clindamycin (Cleocin, Upjohn)

imipenem/cilastatin (Primaxin, Merck)

metronidazole (Flagyl, SCS)

pentamidine (Pentam, Fujisawa)

trimethoprim/sulfamethoxazole (Bactrim, Roche; Septra, Burroughs Wellcome)

vancomycin (Vancocin, Lilly)

(Vancoled, Lederle)

2. **Chemotherapy (Anticancer) Agents**

aldesleukin (Proleukin, Chlron)

bleomycin (Blenoxane, Bristol-Myers Oncology)

carboplatin (Paraplatin, B-M Oncology)

carmustine (BiCNU, B-M Oncology)

cisplatin (Platinol, B-M Oncology)

cyclophosphamide (Cytoxan, B-M Oncology; Neosar, Pharmacia Adria)

cytarabine (Cytosar-U, Upjohn)

dactinomycin (Cosmegen, Merck)

daunorubicin (Cerubidine, Wyeth-Ayerst)

etoposide (VePesid, B-M Oncology)

fluorouracil

idarubicin (Idamycin, Pharmacia Adria)

ifosfamide (IFEX, B-M Oncology)

interferon alfa-2a (Roferon-A, Roche)

interferon alfa-2b (Intron A, Schering)

leucovorin

leuprolide (Lupron, TAP)

lomustine (CeeNU, B-M Oncology)

methotrexate

mitomycin (Mutamycin, B-M Oncology)

mitoxantrone (Novantrone, Lederle)

octreotide (Sandostatin, Sandoz)

pentostatin (Nipent, Parke-Davis)

plicamycin (Mithracin, Miles)

streptozocin (Zanosar, Upjohn)

vinblastine (Velban, Lilly)

vincristine (Oncovin, Lilly)

3. **Electrolytes**

calcium gluconate

magnesium sulfate

potassium chloride

potassium phosphate

sodium bicarbonate

sodium chloride

potassium acetate

sodium acetate

4. **Steroids**

dexamethasone (Decadron, Merck; Hexadrol, Organon)

hydrocortisone (Hydrocortone, Merck; Solu-Cortef, Upjohn)

methylprednisolone (Solu-Medrol, Upjohn)

5. **Cardiovascular Drugs**

dobutamine (Dobutrex, Lilly)

dopamine (Intropin, Du Pont)

isoproterenol (Isuprel, Sanofi Winthrop)

lidocaine (Xylocaine, Astra)

nitroglycerin (Tridil, Du Pont)

nitroprusside (Nipride, Roche)

6. **Antivirals**

acyclovir (Zovirax, Burroughs Wellcome)

foscarnet (Foscavir, Astra)

ganciclovir (Cytovene, Syntex)

interferon alfa-n3 (Alferon N, Purdue Frederick)

vidarabine (Vira-A, Parke-Davis)

zidovudine (Retrovir, Burroughs Wellcome)

7. **Colony-Stimulating Factors**

filgrastim (Neupogen, Amgen)

sargramostim (Leukine, Immunex; Prokine, Hoechst-Roussel)

8. **Immunosuppressives**

azathioprine (Imuran, Burroughs Wellcome)

cyclosporin (Sandimmune, Sandoz)

lymphocyte immune globulin, antithymocyte globulin (Atgam, Upjohn)

muromonab-CD3 (Orthoclone OKT3, Ortho Biotech)

9. **Antinauseants**

granisetron (Kytril, SmithKline Beecham)

ondansetron (Zofran, Cerenex)

10. **Histamine H-2 Antagonists**

cimetidine (Tagamet, SmithKline Beecham)

famotidine (Pepcid, Merck)

ranitidine (Zantac, Glaxo)

11. **Trace Elements**

manganese

chromium

selenium

zinc

copper

12. *Miscellaneous Drugs*

> aminophylline
>
> heparin
>
> immune globulin I.V., human
>
> > (Gamimune, Miles Biological)
> >
> > (Gammar, Armour)
> >
> > (Gammagard, Baxter)
> >
> > (Polygam, American Red Cross)
> >
> > (Sandoglobulin, Sandoz)
>
> multivitamins
>
> oxytocin (Pitocin, Parke-Davis)
>
> insulin, human regular (Humulin, Lilly; Novolin, Novo Nordisk)

The disease or condition for which a drug is used is said to be an *indication* for that drug. For example, penicillin is indicated for infections caused by certain bacteria. In contrast, a *contra-indication* is any condition under which a drug should not be used. For example, penicillin is contraindicated if the patient is allergic to it.

MECHANISMS OF DRUG ACTION

Drugs act or bring about their therapeutic effect in several ways. Some types of action are simple, some are very complex, and others are unknown. Fundamentally, drugs act by altering some physiological process within the body, usually at the cellular level, although the nature of the action is extremely variable.

The cells on which drugs exert their action are known as *target cells*. Target cells have a specific location on which the drug acts, called the *receptor site*. A drug interacts specifically with the receptor site because the two fit together much like a lock and key (figure 3.2).

To be effective, a drug must reach the site where it can act; that is, it must first get into the blood stream to be transported to the site of action. Because there are no barriers to absorption into the blood stream when the I.V. route is used, *distribution* of the drug throughout the body occurs within a few minutes. Reaching the site of action where the drug can combine with the target cells is usually not a concern with I.V. therapy.

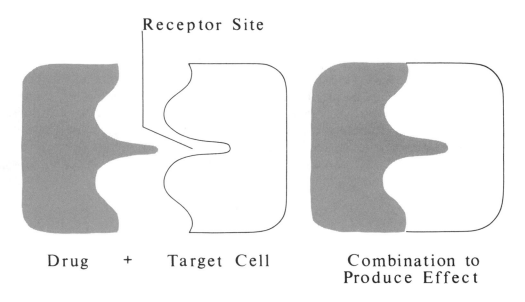

Receptor Site

Drug + Target Cell | Combination to Produce Effect

FIGURE 3.2. INTERACTION OF DRUGS AND TARGET CELLS

The drug is often chemically altered or broken down (*metabolized*) to an inactive form before it leaves the body. Metabolism is one way in which the duration of drug action is limited in the body. Drugs are eliminated (*excreted*) from the body in a variety of ways, the most common being in the urine. Dosage adjustments may be necessary if disease has affected organs responsible for metabolism (e.g., liver) or excretion of a drug (e.g., kidneys).

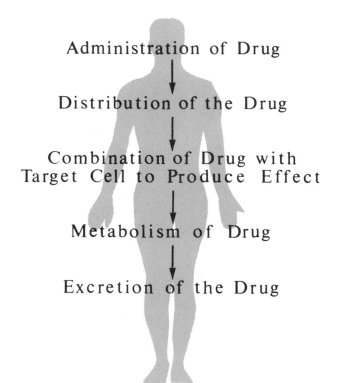

Administration of Drug

Distribution of the Drug

Combination of Drug with
Target Cell to Produce Effect

Metabolism of Drug

Excretion of the Drug

FIGURE 3.3. DRUG TRACED THROUGH THE BODY

FACTORS INFLUENCING DRUG DOSES

The *dose* of a drug is the amount of drug administered at one time. It is usually specified as a certain weight or volume of the drug, although there are many exceptions. (Weights and measures of drugs are discussed in chapter 7.) The recommended dose of a drug to produce the desired effect is known as the *therapeutic dose*. The therapeutic dose lies somewhere between the smallest dose that produces the desired effect (the *minimal effective dose*) and the largest dose that can be safely given (the *maximum safe dose*). If the maximum safe dose is exceeded, adverse or toxic effects may occur; this dose is known as a *toxic dose*. If the minimum effective dose is not achieved, the drug will be ineffective; this dose is called a *subtherapeutic dose*. Figure 3.4 graphically shows the relationship of these terms.

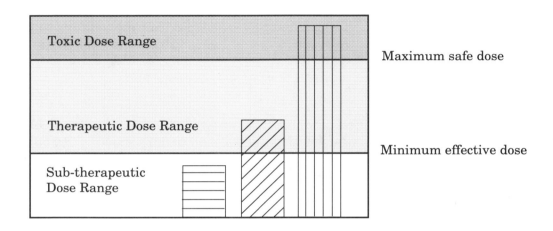

FIGURE 3.4. RELATIONSHIP OF DIFFERENT DOSES

The physician and pharmacist share the responsibility for prescribing medication correctly for an individual patient. This includes the right medication, right dosage form, right dose, and right route of administration. The physician and pharmacist must also make sure that a drug is not contraindicated and that it does not interact with another drug the patient is currently taking. If a question arises about a prescription order, the pharmacist must clarify the point with the physician or nurse as appropriate.

Several factors must be considered when the dose of a drug is prescribed for a patient. Some of these factors can be controlled; others cannot. Following are some of the important factors that influence the dose of a drug for an individual patient.

Body Weight The amount of drug administered in relation to the weight of the patient determines the concentration of drug in the body. The dose of a drug often must increase in proportion to the weight of an individual to achieve the same therapeutic effect. Because body weight varies so greatly among patients, the drug dose should be appropriately adjusted, especially if the patient is notably large or small. Body weight or body surface area is often used as a basis for calculating the dose prescribed, especially in pediatric patients.

Route of Administration This factor was discussed briefly in chapter 2. Because absorption of the drug into the blood circulation varies with the route of administration, the dose may need to be adjusted. Some drugs may be administered only by the I.V. route because they are not absorbed using other routes. Likewise, some drugs may be administered orally when an injectable form of the drug is not available.

Drug Interactions The effectiveness and safety of a drug may be affected by the administration of another drug at the same time. A drug interaction may result in an unintended, adverse effect if the possible combined effects are unknown or are not taken into consideration. Occasionally, the interaction of two drugs can be taken advantage of if one drug magnifies the beneficial effect of the other. In general, known drug-drug or drug-food interactions should be avoided.

Age Besides obvious differences in body weight, very young and very old patients must be given special consideration when drugs and doses are prescribed. Physiological systems in children, especially in infants, may not be mature enough to metabolize or excrete a drug adequately once it is administered. Also, elderly individuals frequently receive a modified dosage because they may respond to drugs in a somewhat different manner because of deteriorating body functions.

Disease The presence of disease may require a dose adjustment of some drugs. Increased severity of a disease frequently requires an increased dose. On the other hand, if the organs involved in metabolism and excretion of a drug are impaired, a smaller dose is usually indicated to prevent the drug from having a magnified effect. For example, patients with renal impairment (i.e., kidney disease) require smaller doses of certain drugs because the kidney does not excrete them at the normal rate.

ADVERSE DRUG REACTIONS

Occasionally, patients have an unwanted and unexpected response to drug therapy that requires intervention on their behalf. Such intervention may consist of discontinuing the drug, changing the dose, treating symptoms of the adverse reaction, or keeping the patient hospitalized longer than intended. An adverse drug reaction may be caused by the drug or by an idiosyncrasy of a specific patient. Adverse drug reactions are tracked by the pharmacy department on an ongoing basis and reported periodically to the P & T committee. Unusual adverse drug reactions should be reported to the drug manufacturer and to the FDA.

When a drug is administered to a patient, three types of responses may occur:

- Desired action—the preventive, diagnostic, or therapeutic effect intended

- Side effects—the undesirable but *predictable* effects that are widely reported and occur in a known percentage of patients

- Adverse drug reactions—the undesirable, yet *unexpected* effects that are not widely reported and occur in only a small percentage of patients

Most drugs have side effects and the potential for adverse drug reactions. These possibilities are usually stated in a package insert under sections covering side effects, precautions, or warnings. Whenever a drug is prescribed, the balance between benefit and risk must always be taken into consideration.

DRUG PACKAGING AND STORAGE

Drugs used in compounding I.V. admixtures are packaged by manufacturers in several different ways (figure 3.5). Liquid drugs are supplied in prefilled syringes, heat-sealed glass containers (*ampules*), or in glass vials sealed with a rubber closure. Powdered drugs are supplied in vials and must be *reconstituted* (dissolved in a suitable liquid) before being added to the I.V. solution. All of these packages are designed to preserve the sterility of their contents. The proper techniques for transferring these drugs to the I.V. solution container are described in chapter 9.

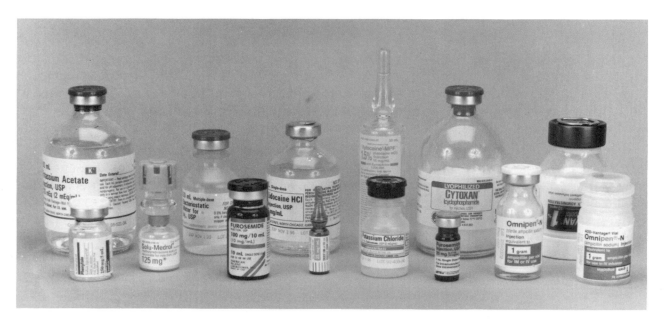

FIGURE 3.5. AMPULES AND VIALS

The label of every drug package includes the following information (figure 3.6):

- The brand name (proprietary, or trademark name) of the drug, if one exists

- The generic name (nonproprietary, or common name) of the drug

- If the drug is in liquid form, the total amount of drug, the total volume of solution, and/or the concentration of the solution

- If the drug is in powder form, the total amount of drug, and possibly directions for reconstitution (also in the package insert)

- If the drug requires a prescription in order to be dispensed, the following statement must appear: "Caution: Federal law prohibits dispensing without prescription"

- The name and address of the manufacturer or distributor

- The manufacturer's or distributor's catalog number for the product

- The lot number, which is a quality control number assigned by the manufacturer

- Precautions specific to the drug, if needed

- An expiration date to indicate a time after which the drug should not be used

- Required storage conditions (e.g., refrigerate)

- A National Drug Code (NDC) number, which identifies a specific drug and package size of a particular manufacturer
- Approved routes of administration

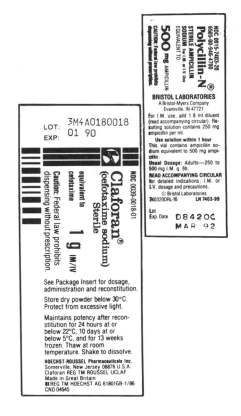

FIGURE 3.6. TYPICAL LABELS ON DRUG PACKAGES

Each drug package contains a package insert providing important information about the drug (figure 3.7). The insert provides a description of the drug, action and uses, dosage and administration, directions for use, precautions and warnings, contraindications, conditions for storage, adverse reactions, and dosage forms available.

Drugs must be stored under specified conditions to protect them from deterioration. Temperature, light, and moisture are the most important factors affecting the potency and stability of drugs. Most drugs should be stored in a cool, dry place. Drugs that must be protected from light are usually packaged in amber-colored ampules or in individual boxes. Some drugs must be refrigerated. Drugs that are supplied in powder form should be refrigerated after reconstitution, even though they may be stored at room temperature prior to that time. Most drugs have a relatively short expiration period after they are reconstituted, so the date and time of reconstitution of a drug should be noted on the vial, along with the initials of the person who reconstituted it.

For Use Only With a Calibrated Infusion Device

Highly Concentrated | Potassium Chloride Injection in Plastic Container

Ready to Use
Viaflex® Plus Container

Description
This Potassium Chloride Injection, is a sterile, nonpyrogenic, highly concentrated, ready-to-use, solution of Potassium Chloride, USP in Water for Injection, USP for electrolyte replenishment in a single dose container for intravenous administration. It contains no antimicrobial agents. Composition, osmolarity, pH and ionic concentration are shown in Table 1.

This Viaflex® Plus plastic container is fabricated from a specially formulated polyvinyl chloride (PL 146® Plastic). Viaflex® containers including Viaflex® Plus containers are made of flexible plastic and are for parenteral use. Viaflex® Plus on the container indicates the presence of a drug additive in a drug vehicle. The amount of water that can permeate from inside the container into the overwrap is insufficient to affect the solution significantly. Solutions in contact with the plastic container can leach out certain of its chemical components in very small amounts within the expiration period, e.g. di-2-ethylhexyl phthalate (DEHP), up to 5 parts per million. However, the safety of the plastic has been confirmed in tests in animals according to USP biological tests for plastic containers as well as by tissue culture toxicity studies.

Clinical Pharmacology
Potassium is the major cation of body cells (160 mEq/liter of intracellular water) and is concerned with the maintenance of body fluid composition and electrolyte balance. Potassium participates in carbohydrate utilization, protein synthesis, and is critical in the regulation of nerve conduction and muscle contraction, particularly in the heart. Chloride, the major extracellular anion, closely follows the metabolism of sodium, and changes in the acid-base of the body are reflected by changes in the chloride concentration.

Normally about 80 to 90% of the potassium intake is excreted in the urine, the remainder in the stools and to a small extent, in the perspiration. The kidney does not conserve potassium well so that during fasting, or in patients on a potassium-free diet, potassium loss from the body continues resulting in potassium depletion. A deficiency of either potassium or chloride will lead to a deficit of the other.

Indications and Usage
Potassium Chloride Injection is indicated in the treatment of potassium deficiency states when oral replacement is not feasible.

This highly concentrated, ready-to-use Potassium Chloride Injection is intended for the maintenance of serum K+ levels and for potassium supplementation in fluid restricted patients. It is also intended for other patients that cannot accommodate additional volumes of fluid associated with potassium solutions of lower concentration.

Contraindications
Potassium Chloride Injection is contraindicted in diseases where high potassium levels may be encountered, and in patients with hyperkalemia, renal failure and in conditions in which potassium retention is present.

Warnings
To avoid potassium intoxication, do not infuse these solutions rapidly.

Administer intravenously only with a calibration infusion device at a slow, controlled rate. (See Dosage and Administration). Whenever possible, administration via a central route is recommended for thorough dilution by the blood stream and avoidance of extravasation.

In patients with renal insufficiency, administration of potassium chloride may cause potassium intoxication and life-threatening hyperkalemia.

The administration of intravenous solutions can cause fluid and/or solute overload resulting in dilution of serum electrolyte concentrations, overhydration, congested states or pulmonary edema. The risk of dilutional states is inversely proportional to the electrolyte concentration. The risk of solute overload causing congested states with peripheral and pulmonary edema is directly proportional to the electrolyte concentration.

Precautions
General
Clinical evaluation and periodic laboratory determinations are necessary to monitor changes in fluid balance, electrolyte concentrations, and acid-base balance during prolonged parenteral therapy or whenever the condition of the patient warrants such evaluation. Significant deviations from normal concentrations may require the use of additional electrolyte supplements, or the use of electrolyte-free dextrose solutions to which individualized electrolyte supplements may be added.

Potassium therapy should be guided primarily by serial electrocardiograms, especially in patients receiving digitalis. Serum potassium levels are not necessarily indicative of tissue potassium levels. Solutions containing potassium should be used with caution in the presence of cardiac disease, particularly in the presence of renal disease, and in such instances, cardiac monitoring is recommended.

Usage in Pregnancy
Pregnancy Category C. Animal reproduction studies have not been conducted with potassium chloride. It is also not known whether potassium chloride can cause fetal harm when administered to a pregnant woman or can affect reproduction capacity. Potassium chloride should be given to a pregnant women only if clearly needed.

Do not administer unless solution is clear and seal is intact.

Adverse Reactions
Reactions which may occur because of the solution or the technique of administration include febrile response, infection at the site of injection, venous thrombosis or phlebitis extending from the site of injection, extravasation, hypervolemia, and hyperkalemia.

Too rapid infusion of hypertonic solutions or highly concentrated potassium chloride solutions may cause local pain and vein irritation. Rate of administration should be adjusted according to tolerance.

Reactions reported with the use of potassium-containing solutions include nausea, vomiting, and abdominal pain and diarrhea. The signs and symptoms of potassium intoxication include paresthesia of the extremities, areflexia, muscular or respiratory paralysis, mental confusion, weakness, hypotension, cardiac arrhythmias, heart block, electrocardiographic abnormalities and cardiac arrest. Potassium deficits results in disruption of neuromuscular function, and intestinal ileus and dilatation.

If an adverse reaction does occur, discontinue the infusion, evaluate the patient, institute appropriate therapeutic countermeasures and save the remainder of the fluid for examination if deemed necessary.

Overdosage
In the event of fluid overload during parenteral therapy, reevaluate the patient's condition, and institute appropriate corrective treatment.

In the event of overdosage with potassium-containing solutions, discontinue the infusion immediately and institute corrective therapy to reduce serum potassium levels.

Treatment of hyperkalemia includes the following:
1. Dextrose Injection, USP, 10% or 25%, containing 10 units of crystalline insulin per 20 grams of dextrose administered intravenously, 300 to 500 mL per hour.
2. Absorption and exchange of potassium using sodium or ammonium cycle cation exchange resin, orally and as retention enema.
3. Hemodialysis and peritoneal dialysis. The use of potassium-containing foods or medications must be eliminated. However, in cases of digitalization, too rapid a lowering of plasma potassium concentration can cause digitalis toxicity.

Dosage and Administration
The dose and rate of administration are dependent upon the specific condition of each patient.

Administer intravenously only with a calibrated infusion device at a slow, controlled rate. Whenever possible, administration via a central route is recommended for thorough dilution by the blood stream and avoidance of extravasation.

Recommended administration rates should not usually exceed 10 mEq/hour or 200 mEq for a 24 hour period if the serum potassium level is greater than 2.5 mEq/liter.

In urgent cases where the serum potassium level is less than 2.0 mEq/liter or where severe hypokalemia is a threat, (serum potassium level less than 2.0 mEq/liter and electrocardiographic changes and/or muscle paralysis) rates up to 40 mEq/hour or 400 mEq over a 24 hour period can be administered very carefully when guided by continuous monitoring of the EKG and frequent serum K+ determinations to avoid hyperkalemia and cardiac arrest.

Parenteral drug products should be inspected visually for particulate matter and discoloration, whenever solution and container permit. Use of a final filter is recommended during administration of all parenteral solutions where possible.

Do not add supplementary medication.

How Supplied
Table 1 shows the available sizes of highly concentrated Potassium Chloride Injection in Viaflex® Plus plastic containers.

Exposure of pharmaceutical products to heat should be minimized. Avoid excessive heat. It is recommended that this product be stored at room temperature (25°C); brief exposure up to 40°C does not affect the product.

Directions for Use of Viaflex® Plus Plastic Container
Do not use plastic containers in series connections. Such use could result in air embolism due to residual air being drawn from the primary container before administration of the fluid from the secondary container is completed.

To Open
Tear overwrap down side at slit and remove solution container. Some opacity of the plastic due to moisture absorption during the sterilization process may be observed. This is normal and does not affect the solution quality or safety. The opacity will diminish gradually. Check for minute leaks by squeezing inner bag firmly. If leaks are found, discard solution as sterility may be impaired. **Do not add supplementary medication.**

Preparation for Administration
1. Suspend container from eyelet support.
2. Remove plastic protector from outlet port at bottom of container.
3. Attach administration set. Refer to complete directions accompanying set.

Table 1

Potassium Chloride Injection mEq Potassium/Container	Composition (g/L) Potassium Chloride, USP (KCl)	Osmolarity (mOsmol/L) (calc) *	pH	Ionic Concentration (mEq/L) Potassium	Chloride	How Supplied Size (mL)	Code	NDC
10 mEq	7.46	200	5 (4 to 8)	100	100	100	2B0826	NDC 0338-0709-48
10 mEq 20 mEq	14.9	400	5 (4 to 8)	200	200	50 100	2B0821 2B0827	NDC 0338-0705-41 NDC 0338-0705-48
30 mEq	22.4	601	5 (4 to 8)	300	300	100	2B0823	NDC 0338-0707-48
20 mEq 40 mEq	29.8	799	5 (4 to 8)	400	400	50 100	2B0822 2B0824	NDC 0338-0703-41 NDC 0338-0703-48

* Normal physiologic osmolarity range is approximately 280 to 310 mOsmol/L. Administration of substantially hypertonic solutions (≥600 mOsmol/L) may cause vein damage.

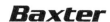

Baxter Healthcare Corporation, I.V. Systems Division, 1425 Lake Cook Road, Deerfield, Illinois 60015

230026   3/91   10M   Printed in U.S.A.

FIGURE 3.7. PACKAGE INSERT

CHAPTER 4

INTRAVENOUS SOLUTIONS

WHY DRUGS ARE ADMINISTERED BY INTRAVENOUS INFUSION

As discussed in chapter 2, I.V. infusions are of two types: continuous and intermittent (or piggyback). Administering medications and fluids by these two methods has several advantages:

1. Continuous infusion provides essential fluid replacement.
2. Continuous infusion keeps the vein open.
3. Intermittent infusion allows the medication to be administered over a longer period of time than with an I.V. push. This allows for greater safety in administering medications that should be injected over a period of several minutes.
4. Intermittent infusion is more dilute than a medication administered by I.V. push, making it less irritating to the vein.
5. The intermittent infusion setup described in chapter 2 allows more efficient use of a nurse's time. Rather than pushing a drug into the vein from a syringe over several minutes, the nurse can turn on the piggyback solution, which will flow in preference to the continuous large-volume solution; when the piggyback solution has been totally infused, infusion of the continuous solution resumes automatically.

CHARACTERISTICS DESIRED IN AN INTRAVENOUS SOLUTION

Intravenous solutions must possess certain characteristics, some of which can be seen by visual inspection and some of which cannot.

Clarity The solution must be _clear_ (not to be confused with colorless) to indicate that the drug is completely dissolved. One notable exception is I.V. fat emulsions that look similar to milk. The solution must also be _free of visible particulate matter_ such as fibers or rubber cores from vials.

Sterility Sterility, equal pH, and isotonicity are essential characteristics of I.V. solutions that cannot be assessed visually. _Sterility_ is the freedom from bacteria and other microorganisms. Solutions for injection must be sterile, which is not a relative term; an item is either sterile or not sterile. It is incorrect to refer to something as being partially sterile. When drugs are added to I.V. solutions, good aseptic technique must be used to maintain the sterility of solutions, drugs, and supplies.

_pH_ The term _pH_ is used to describe the degree of acidity of a solution (figure 4.1). pH values range from 0 to 14, with values below 7 representing greater _acidity_ and values above 7 representing less acidity (greater _alkalinity_). A solution having a pH of 7 is neither acidic nor alkaline; it is neutral.

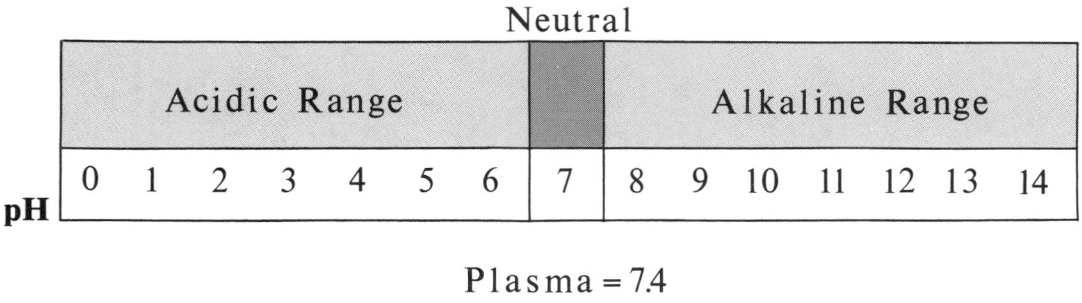

Neutral

pH	Acidic Range								Alkaline Range						
	0	1	2	3	4	5	6	7	8	9	10	11	12	13	14

Plasma = 7.4

FIGURE 4.1. pH SCALE

Plasma is slightly alkaline, with a normal pH of about 7.4. Because many complex processes occur in the body to maintain this pH value, an effort should be made to provide an I.V. solution that does not vary significantly from the normal pH. Of course, there are situations in which this becomes a secondary consideration because acidic or alkaline solutions may be indicated and even lifesaving.

Isotonicity Isotonic I.V. solutions minimize patient discomfort and damage to red blood cells. Fluid inside the cells contains dissolved substances such as sugars and salts. The cell is surrounded by a wall or membrane that permits fluid, but not the dissolved substances, to pass freely. The membrane is described as a *semipermeable membrane* because it is readily permeable only by the fluid (figure 4.2).

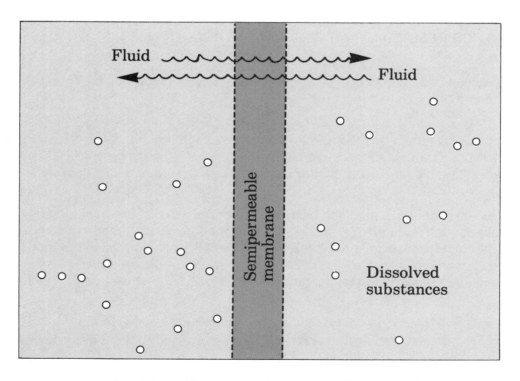

FIGURE 4.2. DIFFUSION ACROSS A SEMIPERMEABLE MEMBRANE

If the red blood cells are in a solution containing a concentration of dissolved substances lower than that of the cells, water moves into the red blood cells, causing the cells to swell. On the other hand, if red blood cells are in a solution that contains a greater concentration of dissolved substances than in the cells, water moves out of the cells and into the solution, causing the cells to shrink. It should be noted that the fluid always moves toward the higher concentration of dissolved substances in an effort to equalize the two concentrations.

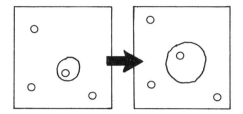 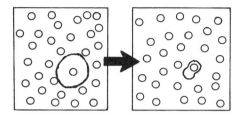

Red blood cell <u>swells</u> when the surrounding fluid has a <u>lower</u> concentration of dissolved substances.

Red blood cell <u>shrinks</u> when the surrounding fluid has a <u>higher</u> concentration of dissolved substances.

FIGURE 4.3. EFFECT OF SOLUTIONS WITH DIFFERENT CONCENTRATIONS ON RED CELLS

A solution containing a concentration of dissolved substances less than red blood cells is known as a *hypotonic* solution. A solution that contains a higher concentration of dissolved substances than red blood cells is known as a *hypertonic* solution. If the concentration of a solution is the same as red blood cells, the solution is described as *isotonic*. When practical, I.V. solutions should be as close to isotonic as possible. These solutions are shown graphically in figure 4.4.

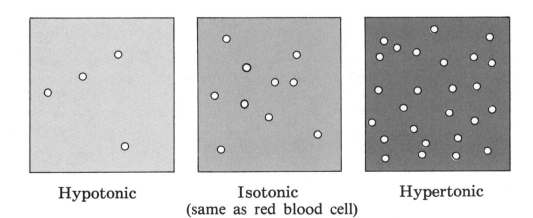

Hypotonic   Isotonic   Hypertonic
                 (same as red blood cell)

FIGURE 4.4. RELATIVE SOLUTION CONCENTRATIONS OF DISSOLVED SUBSTANCES IN DIFFERENT SOLUTIONS

Stinging caused by a hypertonic or hypotonic solution is not experienced with an isotonic solution. A good reference point to remember is that 0.9% sodium chloride injection and 5% dextrose injection are both approximately isotonic.

VOLUME OF SOLUTION INFUSED

The volume of I.V. solution infused depends upon the condition of the patient. For patients whose fluid intake is restricted, the volume of fluid infused needs to be minimized. Other patients may require a large volume of solution to replace fluid loss due to their disease condition. The volume of solution, as well as the solution itself, is prescribed by the physician. The most common sizes of I.V. solutions are 1,000, 500, 250, 100, and 50 milliliters (mL or ml).

STORAGE CONDITIONS FOR SOLUTIONS

I.V. solutions should be stored at room temperature or in a cool place. Care should be taken to avoid freezing large-volume parenterals (250 to 1,000 mL) in glass because this will cause the fluid to expand, cracking or breaking the bottle. This is not a danger with I.V. bags. Cold temperatures may cause some concentrated solutions (e.g., mannitol) to precipitate. Likewise, solutions should not be stored at high temperatures, particularly if they contain drugs, because such storage may accelerate decomposition of the drug. Storage instructions are included as part of the labeling on the I.V. solution container.

TYPES OF SOLUTIONS USED

Many different solutions are commercially available; however, combinations and variations of three standard solutions are most frequently used in I.V. admixtures. The three standard solutions are sodium chloride injection, dextrose injection, and Ringer's injection. Components of these solutions are compared in figure 4.5.

The most frequently used strengths of sodium chloride are 0.9%, 0.45%, and 0.2%. A 0.9% sodium chloride injection is often referred to as *normal saline* or isotonic saline. Sodium chloride solutions are used primarily as a source of fluid and electrolytes.

Dextrose injection (also referred to as glucose injection) is most frequently used in a 5% concentration. Higher concentrations are available, but because they are too hypertonic to be infused directly, they are used in compounding specialized solutions. Dextrose solutions are used primarily as a source of fluid and carbohydrates for nutrition. Various combinations of different strengths of sodium chloride and dextrose solutions are also available, e.g., 5% dextrose and 0.45% sodium chloride injection, or 5% dextrose and 0.2% sodium chloride injection.

Ringer's injection, which contains the primary electrolytes found in plasma, can be modified by the addition of sodium lactate to produce lactated Ringer's injection. Ringer's solutions are used primarily for fluid replacement and as a source of electrolytes. Ringer's injection and lactated Ringer's injection do not contain therapeutic amounts of potassium and calcium. Correction of potassium and calcium deficits is accomplished best by the addition of more suitable additives for this purpose, i.e., potassium chloride or calcium gluconate in therapeutic amounts.

INTRAVENOUS SOLUTION	DEXTROSE HYDROUS	ELECTROLYTES (mEq/L)					TONICITY DESIGNATION	pH
		Sodium	Potassium	Calcium	Chloride	Lactate		
5% Dextrose Inj.	50	—	—	—	—	—	Isotonic	3.5-6.5
10% Dextrose Inj.	100	—	—	—	—	—	Hypertonic	3.5-6.5
0.9% Sodium Chloride Inj.	—	154	—	—	154	—	Isotonic	4.5-7.0
0.45% Sodium Chloride Inj.	—	77	—	—	77	—	Hypotonic	4.5-7.0
5% Dextrose and 0.9% Sodium Chloride Inj.	50	154	—	—	154	—	Hypertonic	3.5-6.5
5% Dextrose and 0.45% Sodium Chloride Inj.	50	77	—	—	77	—	Hypertonic	3.5-6.5
5% Dextrose and 0.2% Sodium Chloride Inj.	50	34	—	—	34	—	Isotonic	3.5-6.5
Ringer's Inj.	—	147	4	5	156	—	Isotonic	5.0-7.5
Lactated Ringer's Inj.	—	130	4	3	109	28	Isotonic	6.0-7.5
Lactated Ringer's and Dextrose Inj.	50	130	4	3	109	28	Hypertonic	4.0-6.5

FIGURE 4.5. COMPONENTS OF MOST COMMONLY USED I.V. SOLUTIONS

MAINTENANCE THERAPY AND REPLACEMENT THERAPY

Maintenance therapy refers to the patient's routine daily fluid and electrolyte needs. A patient whose oral intake is restricted must be given fluid and electrolytes intravenously to replace body water lost through normal body respiration, perspiration, urination, etc. A patient may receive as many as three liters (L) of maintenance solution each day.

On the other hand, *replacement therapy* refers to restoring acute losses of fluid and electrolytes from surgery, trauma, burns, or shock. Replacement solutions should closely approximate the electrolyte content of the body fluids lost, thus they are quite variable.

CHAPTER 5

INTRAVENOUS ADMIXTURE INCOMPATIBILITIES

INCIDENCE OF INCOMPATIBILITIES

An I.V. admixture is said to be *incompatible* when the prescribed drugs cannot be combined safely and satisfactorily. The incompatibility may be between two drugs or between a drug and the I.V. solution. The incidence of incompatibilities is relatively low when compared to the number of I.V. admixtures prepared, but the possibility of an unexpected or undesirable combination always exists. If an incompatibility goes undetected, the patient may not receive the full therapeutic effect of the medication. Even worse, an incompatibility may lead to an adverse effect on the patient.

TYPES OF INCOMPATIBILITIES

Some incompatibilities result in a physical change that is easily recognizable. This change may be a change in color, evolution of a gas, development of a haze, or formation of solid particles that settle out of solution (i.e., *precipitate*). These are the most obvious incompatibilities to detect because they can be seen.

Other incompatibilities cannot be visually recognized. Two drugs can react to cause the degradation of one or both. These incompatibilities are not detected visually, but they can be confirmed by analytical methods.

Although a change in color of a solution, evolution of a gas, or formation of a precipitate may signal cause for concern about potential incompatibility, these types of physical change sometimes are expected and are not a problem. For example, variations in color of imipenem-cilastatin or dobutamine do not affect potency. When ceftazidime is reconstituted, carbon dioxide gas is released and positive pressure develops. Accumulated gases should be expressed from the syringe or vented from the vial before administration. The precipitate that forms when paclitaxel is refrigerated dissolves at room temperature. This points to the need for a pharmacist to be familiar with the literature and to exercise professional judgment in providing safe, effective drug therapy to patients.

FACTORS AFFECTING COMPATIBILITY AND STABILITY

Many factors may affect the compatibility and/or stability of drugs in I.V. admixtures. Some of the most common factors are described below.

pH The most common cause of incompatibilities is combining two drugs that require conflicting pH values of the final solution for their own stability. If the pH of an admixture is unsuitable for one of the drugs, that drug either degrades or precipitates. Care must be taken, especially when a drug with a low pH is combined with a drug having a high pH. An example is the combination of aminophylline and vitamin B complex with C. Aminophylline has a pH of 8.0 to 9.0, whereas the vitamin preparation has an acidic pH. The high pH of the resulting solution destroys vitamin activity.

Ticarcillin-clavulanate, dobutamine, ondansetron, nitroglycerin, and carmustine are each incompatible with sodium bicarbonate, which has an alkaline pH.

Complexation An example of complexation is the combination of tetracycline with a calcium-containing drug. The chemical complex formed between tetracycline and calcium reduces the antibacterial activity of the tetracycline. Thus, solutions containing calcium should be avoided with tetracycline.

Some drugs interact with aluminum, causing a problem in preparation and administration because most needles are made of aluminum. For example, cisplatin-AQ should not be used with needles, I.V. sets, or filters containing aluminum.

Light Exposure of some drugs to light may destroy or reduce the potency of the drug. Amphotericin B, cisplatin, and metronidazole must be protected from light to maintain their potency.

Dilution The concentration of a drug in solution may be a factor in its compatibility with other drugs. A common problem is the mixing of electrolytes in preparing parenteral nutrition solutions. However, the problem can be avoided by assuring that the electrolytes in question are properly diluted before they are combined. Up to 15 milliequivalents (mEq) of calcium can be added to a liter of solution containing up to 30 mEq of phosphate without precipitating. Higher concentrations of either drug, however, result in precipitation.

Time Most drugs degrade in a relatively short time when placed in an I.V. solution. Similarly, many incompatibilities are not instantaneous, but develop over time.

I.V. Solution Some drugs require specific solutions (diluents) for reconstitution and further dilution. For example, amphotericin B must be reconstituted with sterile water for injection without a bacteriostatic agent and then further diluted only with 5% dextrose injection. Amphotericin B is not compatible with normal saline. Not only is the solution designated to be 5% dextrose injection, but the pH must be above 4.2.

Some drugs are packaged with a specific diluent for use in reconstitution. For example, the diluent for immune globulin is supplied by the manufacturer with specific directions for reconstitution and dilution. Preparation time may be prolonged from 20 minutes with the diluent supplied to 75 and 135 minutes when 3% and 6% immune globulin, respectively, are reconstituted with a 5% dextrose injection. In addition, the diluent and product should be warmed to room temperature before reconstitution, and shaking should be avoided, as it causes foaming.

Temperature The degradation of a drug in solution may be regarded as a chemical reaction. Because heat increases the rate of most chemical reactions, solutions are in most cases more stable at refrigerated temperatures than at room temperature. Cefazolin, once it has been reconstituted in a vial, is stable for 24 hours at room temperature, but for 96 hours under refrigeration. Some drugs, however, should not be refrigerated. Metronidazole should not be refrigerated because it causes mannitol in the formulation to precipitate.

Some drugs can be frozen after reconstitution and stored for prolonged periods. For example, cefazolin is stable for at least 12 weeks when frozen at -20° C. Ampicillin is an unusual drug with respect to temperature. It is more stable at refrigerated temperatures than at room temperature, but less stable at frozen temperatures than at refrigerated temperatures. For this reason, ampicillin should not be frozen for purposes of prolonging the stability of reconstituted solutions. It is recommended that many drugs not be frozen, either because freezing has not been investigated or it results in a problem. For example, ganciclovir, trimethoprim/sulfamethoxazole, and impipenem-cilastatin should not be frozen.

Buffer Capacity The buffer capacity of a solution is the ability of that solution to resist a change in pH when either an acidic or alkaline substance is added to it. Many drugs contain buffers to increase their stability. In general, I.V. solutions do not have high buffer capacities. Thus, when a drug with a high buffer capacity is added to a common I.V. solution such as 5% dextrose injection, the pH of the resulting solution is close to that of the drug additive. Important exceptions are I.V. solutions that contain lactates and acetates, both of which have a relatively high buffer capacity. Thus, the pH of these solutions does not change as easily, making them more prone to compatibility problems.

Penicillin G may be added to 5% dextrose injection even though the pH of the dextrose solution may be 4.0 and penicillin G is not stable at that pH. However, penicillin G contains a citrate buffer that provides a final pH of 6.0 to 6.5 when added to 5% dextrose injection. The 5% dextrose injection has a very low buffer capacity; that is, it is unable to resist the change in pH when the buffer in penicillin G is added.

Order of Mixing The order in which drugs are added to the solution may be a factor in compatibility. Drugs that are in concentrated solutions may react to form a precipitate, whereas both drugs in diluted solutions may be combined satisfactorily. In preparation of parenteral nutrition solutions, electrolytes such as calcium and magnesium are commonly prescribed with phosphates, creating a compounding problem if not done correctly. By adding the diluted electrolytes last and mixing well after each addition, the electrolytes are well diluted when they come into contact with each other, and the chance of precipitation is minimized.

When compounding all-in-one parenteral nutrition solutions (discussed in chapter 10), the order of mixing is also critical. These complex admixtures consist of a fat emulsion, a dextrose solution, and an amino acid solution. Mixing should start with the fat; then the amino acid is added; and finally the dextrose. The important concept is to avoid adding the dextrose directly to the fat, because it will break the emulsion, causing it to separate.

Plastic In addition to drug-drug and drug-solution incompatibilities, some drugs are incompatible with plastic I.V. bags and administration sets. This is especially true of polyvinyl chloride (PVC) plastic. The drug may leach plasticizers out of the bag or set, or the drug may adhere to the bag or set, making it unavailable for its intended therapeutic effect. It is recommended that carmustine be used in glass containers only. Cyclosporin and paclitaxel should always be mixed in non-PVC bags and administered in non-PVC tubing. Interferons are not stable in polypropylene syringes designed for use in ambulatory infusion pumps.

Small amounts of albumin can sometimes be added to the admixture if the drug adheres to the I.V. bag because it is preferentially adsorbed to the surface of the plastic. However, this is an expensive practice and the advantages of doing so should be carefully considered. Albumin (1 mL/50 mL 0.9% sodium chloride injection) can be added to solutions of sargramostim to prevent adsorption to the plastic of the I.V. delivery system.

Filters Final filters (discussed in chapter 2) represent a possible problem in effective delivery of the drug to the patient, even though technically the problem may not be a compatibility or stability issue. The addition of an in-line filter causes an 86% to 94% reduction in the delivered concentration of nitroglycerin. Cisplatin-AQ should not be used with filters containing aluminum (common paper filters do not contain aluminum). On the other hand, it is recommended that some drugs be administered with an in-line filter; e.g., ganciclovir must be infused using a 5- or 0.22-micron filter. Again, knowledge about the safe and effective preparation and administration of each drug is a professional responsibility of the pharmacist.

SOURCES OF INFORMATION

The most frequently used sources of information on incompatibilities are manufacturers' drug package inserts, incompatibility charts, published articles, and reference books.

Package Inserts A package insert generally contains little incompatibility information, especially for new drugs. The package insert is developed by the manufacturer and approved by the FDA when the drug is marketed. At that point, few studies have been done to determine with which agents the new drug can be safely combined. It is also an expensive and time-consuming process to add such information to the package insert voluntarily at a later time.

The package insert, however, often provides important information that enables a pharmacist to make an informed judgment as to the compatibility of a drug combination. For example, a package insert may specify the pH range over which the drug is most stable or the stability of the drug once it has been added to an I.V. solution. Some package inserts do provide valuable information by actually listing specific drugs that have been tested and shown to be compatible or incompatible with that drug.

Incompatibility Charts Incompatibility charts are available that list drugs that can and cannot be mixed in particular solutions. Some charts list drugs horizontally across the top and vertically down one side. One drug is found in the top list and the other drug in the side list; then the two constituents of the admixture are followed along the lines from the top and the side until they intersect. A notation in the space where the lines intersect denotes whether or not the mixture is compatible. The major limitation of some charts is that they do not state why a particular mixture is incompatible, providing little, if any, information on the relative conditions (e.g., pH, concentration) under which the tests were conducted.

The *Guide to Parenteral Admixtures* (see References, appendix A) is one example of a chart that provides information beyond whether or not two drugs are compatible. The *Guide*, a page from which is shown in figure 5.1, may specify the concentration of the constituents and reasons that a drug combination is not compatible. An important advantage to this reference is that the data are continually updated by supplements. To use the guide:

1. Select the chart for one of the drug constituents under its generic name.
2. Find the other drug on the list down the side and follow that line horizontally across to the space under the solution prescribed.
3. At this intersection, a notation is made as to the compatibility of the admixture solution— whether the mixture is compatible (C), incompatible (X), conflicting data exist (𝒞) or no data exist (blank).

Literature and Books Information on incompatibilities can often be found in articles in professional journals and in reference books dealing specifically with the subject. The *American Journal of Health-System Pharmacy* (formerly the *American Journal of Hospital Pharmacy*) frequently has detailed research articles on intravenous incompatibilities. Two reference books that are very useful are the

AMINOPHYLLINE (cont'd-2)	Unspec.	D 5 W	D 10 W	D 5 LR	D 5 ¼S	D 5 ½S	D 5 NS	D 5 R	LR	R	Sod Cl 0.9	Sod Lac
Bretylium Tosylate		#									#	
#Bretylium (1 mg/ml?) and aminophylline, 1 mg/ml, physically compatible for 48 hours (672).												
Brompheniramine Maleate	ℂ*											
*Physically compatible in direct admixture, except if more than 1 ml aminophylline used (89).												
Calcium Chloride							X					
Calcium Gluconate	C											
Cefazolin Sodium		*									C	
500 mg aminophylline physically compatible with 1 Gm cefazolin in 1 liter normal saline at 5°C or room temperature for 24 hours (167).												
*When 1 Gm cefazolin added to Buretrol with solution of 1 Gm aminophylline in 1 liter D5W solution became amber color (259).												
Cefoperazone Sodium												
When cefoperazone, premixed 2 Gm in D5W, was piggybacked into a solution of aminophylline, 1 Gm in 1000 ml D5W, there was no visual evidence of incompatibility (1029).												
Cefotetan Disodium												
In mixture of cefotetan with aminophylline, 250 mg/10 ml, the mixture was compatible and cefotetan stable for at least 24 hours at room temperature and light; infusion fluid not noted (1193).												
► **Ceftazidime**												
Ceftazidime, 40 mg/ml, with theophylline, 1.6 mg/ml, in NS or D5W, via a simulated Y-site technique, was compatible for up to 2 hours. However, using a simulated constant infusion method, ceftazidime, 2 mg/ml or 6 mg/ml, mixed with theophylline, 0.8 mg/ml or 1.6 mg/ml in NS or D5W, was physically and chemically incompatible (1275).												
Cephalothin Sodium	X	X	X	X	X	X	X	X	X	X	X	X
Cephalothin unstable at high pH.												
Also incompatible in 20% Dextrose in Water.												
Cephapirin Sodium	*	#	X	#	#	*	*	*	*	§	*	
*Compatible for 24 hours; # compatible for 8 hours, X excessive loss of cephapirin activity at 4 hours (also noted in D20W); § compatible for 4 hours (192).												
Cephradine (Velosef for Injection)	*											
*1 Gm cephradine and 500 mg aminophylline physically compatible in 250 mg D5W (415).												
Chloramphenicol Sodium Succinate	ℂ*	X	X	X	ℂ*	X	X	X	X	X	X	
Incompatible notations in grid derived from Ref. 13. More recent observation (331) reports no physical evidence of incompatibility when 125 mg aminophylline and 500 mg chloramphenicol were admixed in 500 ml D5W or D 5 / 1/2S (in Viaflex containers) and observed for 12 hours. Also incompatible in D20W.												
Chlorpromazine Hydrochloride	§											
§Chlorpromazine 50 mg (2 ml) plus aminophylline 500 mg (20 ml) in 1000 ml D5W formed bluish precipitate (211).												
Cibenzoline Succinate	#										#	
#Cibenzoline 2 mg/ml and aminophylline 10 mg/ml visually compatible in D5W or NS for at least 24 hours at room temperature (899).												

FIGURE 5.1. GUIDE TO PARENTERAL ADMIXTURES

Handbook on Injectable Drugs and the *American Hospital Formulary Service, Drug Information*. All three are published by the American Society of Health-System Pharmacists,Bethesda, MD.

Many pharmacy departments maintain a file of published articles to provide detailed information from the primary literature that would not otherwise be readily available. This practice has been carried one step further in some pharmacies that have established index card files with information on each drug condensed from journal articles and other sources. This filing system permits ready access to information when needed. Alternatively, some articles republished periodically provide similar compatibility and stability information, e.g., *Injectable Medications 1994* (see References, appendix A). Some pharmacy computer systems screen for I.V. admixture incompatibilities as well as drug interactions, alerting the pharmacist or pharmacy technician at the time the order is entered into the computer.

Electronic Databases Pharmacies commonly use electronic databases on CD-ROM to access information quickly. These databases, such as Micromedex (Denver, Colorado), contain information on incompatibilities and stability within each drug monograph described. These types of databases have several advantages over printed references: (1) they are updated frequently; (2) they are accessible by any person able to access the computer network regardless of their location; and (3) they take up less space.

MINIMIZING INCOMPATIBILITIES

Incompatibilities can be minimized by following a few general guidelines whenever possible:

1. Use solutions promptly after preparation in order to assure administration of the most stable product, since the degradation of many drugs is time related. If freshly prepared admixtures cannot be used immediately, they should be refrigerated.
2. Minimize the number of drugs added to one solution. As the number of drug additives increases, the possibility of incompatibilities increases geometrically. When more than two drugs are combined in a solution, it is difficult to find adequate information about potential compatibility of the resultant admixture.
3. Check incompatibility references closely if one of the drugs has a very high or very low pH. Because most drugs are acidic, their combination with a drug having a very high pH, such as sodium bicarbonate or aminophylline, is more likely to result in an incompatibility.
4. Check incompatibility references closely when one additive is a drug containing calcium, magnesium, or phosphate, because these substances cause precipitation of many drugs and each other.
5. Check incompatibility references closely if one of the drugs or the I.V. solution contains an acetate or lactate (these substances have a buffering capacity).

RESPONSIBILITY FOR ELIMINATING INCOMPATIBILITIES

Although physicians and pharmacists have a shared responsibility for selecting the most appropriate medication for each patient, pharmacists are best qualified to assure the compatibility of an admixture. Frequently, the I.V. solution is not specified when intermittent (piggyback) drugs are prescribed, leaving it to the pharmacist to select the one most appropriate.

If an incompatible drug combination is prescribed, the pharmacist has a professional and legal responsibility to correct the situation by clarifying questions with the physician or nurse as appropriate. The pharmacist should be prepared to provide an explanation of why the admixture is incompatible, a recommendation of alternative drug therapy, alternative methods of administering the drugs to avoid their mixing, or other possible solutions to the problem. A practical solution to the problem often is changing the I.V. infusion setup to keep the two incompatible drugs separated.

CHAPTER 6

THE PRESCRIPTION AND PRESCRIPTION TERMINOLOGY

A *prescription* is an order by a licensed practitioner, as defined by state law, for the preparation and administration of a medication for a specific patient. Because nearly all prescriptions for I.V. admixtures are written by physicians, that frame of reference is used throughout this manual. Prescriptions or medication orders are usually written by the physician on a special form provided by the hospital or health care organization. In some instances, the prescription may be given verbally to a pharmacist or nurse, in which case it must be recorded in writing immediately and countersigned by the physician, usually within 24 hours, depending on the organization's policy. Verbal orders are usually restricted to emergencies or situations in which the physician is contacted by phone.

PARTS OF A PRESCRIPTION

Although the manner in which physicians write prescriptions varies, each prescription consists of the same essential parts:

- Patient identification
- Date
- Name, strength, and amount of each medication
- Directions for administration
- Physician's signature

Figure 6.1 represents a typical prescription written on a physician's order form for a hospitalized patient. Prescriptions written for outpatients are somewhat different in format, but consist of the same elements listed above. Care should be taken to see that all essential parts of the prescription are complete and appropriate:

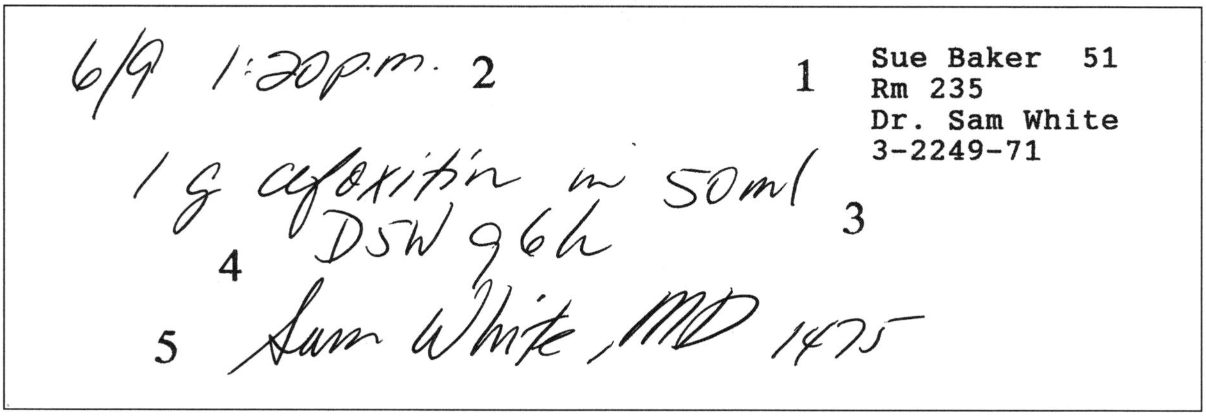
6/9 1:20p.m. 2
1 Sue Baker 51
Rm 235
Dr. Sam White
3-2249-71
1 g cefoxitin in 50ml 3
4 D5W q6h
5 Sam White, MD 1475

FIGURE 6.1. TYPICAL PRESCRIPTION

1. The patient's name, room number, and hospital number are necessary to assure that the patient is properly identified and that the completed admixture is delivered to the correct location. In many hospitals, this information is prestamped on the physician's order form by the unit secretary or clerk in the patient care area.
2. The date, and preferably the time of day, should be on the prescription.
3. The name, strength, and amount of each medication must be specified. The medication may be identified by the generic name, brand name, or an abbreviation.
4. Directions for proper administration of the medication are necessary for the nurse to follow and to instruct the pharmacy as to when the doses must be prepared.
5. The physician's signature must be on each prescription, preferably along with a pager number. If the prescription is telephoned to a nurse or pharmacist, the physician's name should be signed along with the name of the person taking the verbal order. The physician must countersign the verbal order within a specified number of hours—usually less than 24 hours.

LEGIBILITY OF PRESCRIPTIONS

Every prescription or medication order should be understood completely before it is prepared and dispensed because every word and abbreviation is meaningful. To assume that any part of the order is not important because it is illegible can lead to serious errors. Whenever there is the least doubt about the legibility of a prescription or the intention of the prescriber, the pharmacist must resolve the issue by contacting the physician or nurse as appropriate. The legibility of a prescription depends on the experience of the reader as well as on the handwriting of the physician.

ABBREVIATIONS USED WITH ADMIXTURE PRESCRIPTIONS

The following lists include many of the abbreviations commonly used in admixture orders. Abbreviations are not recommended because of possible misinterpretation leading to medication errors, but they are nevertheless widely used.

Abbreviations Related to Schedules

I.V.—intravenous
d—day
q—every, each
qd—every day, daily
qod—every other day
bid—twice a day
tid—3 times a day
qid—4 times a day
h—hour

q(2)h—every (two) hours
npo—nothing by mouth
tko—to keep open
ko—keep open
kvo—keep vein open
PB—piggyback
stat—immediately, at once
prn—as needed, as necessary

Abbreviations Related to Medications

K—potassium
Ca—calcium
Mg—magnesium
Cl—chloride
SO_4—sulfate
HCO_3—bicarbonate
PO_4—phosphate
Na—sodium

W—water
D—dextrose (glucose)
D5W—5% dextrose injection
NS—normal saline (0.9% sodium
chloride injection)
LR—lactated Ringer's injection
TPN—total parenteral nutrition
PN—parenteral nutrition
TNA—total nutrient admixture

Abbreviations Related to Dosage

L—liter
mL—milliliter
cc—cubic centimeter
mEq—milliequivalent
mM—millimole
U—unit

g—gram
mg—milligram
mcg—microgram
µg—microgram
gtt—drop

Following are examples of typical prescriptions with their interpretation.

Example 1

1/30 9⁰⁰ A.m.

John Barrington   23
Rm 739
Dr. George Townson
4-10952-6

Dobutamine 250 mg/L D5W
over 12 h
George Townson, M.D.
T/o M. Shirk, RN

Interpretation: This prescription is for a 23-year-old patient, John Barrington, who is in room 739. The admixture, telephoned to M. Shirk, RN, by Dr. George Townson, at 9 a.m. Jan. 30, is 250 mg of dobutamine added to 1L of 5% dextrose injection and administered over a period of 12 hours, or 84 mL per hour.

Example 2

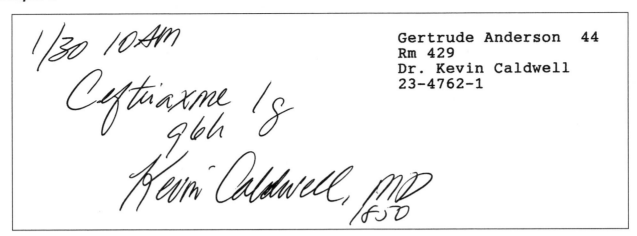

1/30 10AM

Ceftriaxone 1g
q6h

Kevin Caldwell, MD

Gertrude Anderson 44
Rm 429
Dr. Kevin Caldwell
23-4762-1

Interpretation: This prescription is for 44-year-old Gertrude Anderson in room 429 (hospital number 23-4762-1). Dr. Kevin Caldwell wrote the prescription at 10 a.m. Jan. 30. It is for 1g of ceftriaxone every six hours. The diluent and the exact method of administration is not specified, which is common practice. It is generally interpreted that this type of medication, an antibiotic, would be given as an intermittent piggyback infusion over about 20 minutes unless specified otherwise or not recommended in the package insert. Some antibiotics, e.g., gentamicin, are recommended to be given over a longer period of time. The pharmacist would select the most appropriate diluent—in this case, probably 50 mL of D5W. A 50-mL piggyback bag adds less fluid volume than 100-mL bags over four doses per day. This may or may not be an important consideration, depending on the patient. Piggyback bags are available as D5W or NS; D5W is the usual choice because it avoids the sodium present in NS.

Example 3

9/30 2:00 p.m.

40 mEq KCl
1000 mL D5/.45 at 125 mL/hr.
x 8 h post op
Then KO w/D5W

Matthew Johnson, MD

Ralph Martin 42
Rm 120
4-10937-4

Interpretation: This prescription for Ralph Martin in room 120 was written by Dr Matthew Johnson at 2 p.m. Sept. 30. The prescription is for 40 mEq of potassium chloride to be added to 1L of 5% dextrose and 0.45% sodium chloride injection to be infused postoperatively at a rate of 125 mL per hour, for eight hours. Then a solution of 5% dextrose injection will be hung and administered at a rate to keep the vein open.

Example 4

```
2/21  9⁰⁰ AM                      Betty Appel    56
                                  Rm 532
                                  9-177-241

      2000 cc TPN soln daily
      4.25 % Travasol
      20 %   Dextrose
      ⁺ḡ Ca Gluconate      ⁺ḡ MgSO₄
      20 mEq KCl, 50 mEq NaCl   10 mM
                                 K Phosph.
              Fred Gordon MD
```

Interpretation: This prescription is for a parenteral nutrition solution for Betty Appel in room 532. Dr. Fred Gordon wrote the prescription at 9 a.m. Feb. 21. Two liters of parenteral nutrition solution are to be administered daily for an unspecified period. Each 2,000 mL should contain 4.25% Travasol injection, 20% dextrose injection, 1g of calcium gluconate, 1g of magnesium sulfate, 20 mEq of potassium chloride, 50 mEq of sodium chloride, and 10 mM of potassium phosphate. Because this preparation is not commercially available, numerous calculations must be done before the prescription can be prepared. Parenteral nutrition solutions are usually prescribed on a daily basis, rather than a per-bag basis, because it is easier to evaluate and prescribe the total daily intake of calories, electrolytes, grams of nitrogen, etc. Compounding one 2,000-mL bag per day is also easier than compounding two 1,000-mL bags in the pharmacy. Automated compounding machines make calculations and compounding associated with parenteral nutrition solutions much easier, faster, and more accurate than manual methods. Preparation of parenteral nutrition solutions is discussed in chapter 10.

FORMULARY CONSIDERATIONS

Both pharmacists and technicians must be familiar with how a formulary system works in their organization and which drugs the pharmacy and therapeutics (P & T) committee has included in the formulary (this topic was discussed in chapter 3). The selection of formulary drugs should be based on evaluation of their effectiveness, safety, and cost. The committee tries to minimize duplication of the same or similar medications.

Drugs generally are listed in the formulary according to their generic names. Thus, only one brand of a particular drug is stocked in the pharmacy and dispensed on all orders for that drug, regardless of whether it is prescribed by its generic name or one of its trade names. Different brands of the same drug are considered to be identical with respect to their active components and are referred to as *generic equivalents*. For example, the antibiotic ampicillin is included in the formulary by its generic name and only one brand of ampicillin is stocked in the pharmacy. That product is used on all orders for that drug, whether it is prescribed as ampicillin or as one of several brand names available. One ampicillin product is considered to be generically equivalent to all the others.

In order to minimize duplication of similar medications in the formulary, the P & T committee may consider two drugs that are chemically different, but pharmacologically very similar, as *therapeutic equivalents*. The committee generally sets forth policies on how one medication may be dispensed for another if the two have been determined to be therapeutic equivalents. For example, the antinausea drugs ondansetron and granisetron are very similar in comparable doses. In order to minimize therapeutic duplications in the formulary, only one may be included, at least as the preferred agent. The committee may give the pharmacist authority to dispense ondansetron and granisetron interchangeably as therapeutic equivalents within specific guidelines. Thus, when pharmacists and pharmacy technicians interpret prescription orders they must know which medications are routinely stocked in the hospital as formulary agents, the generic equivalents for each drug, and any therapeutic equivalents the pharmacy is authorized to dispense.

CHAPTER 7

CALCULATIONS INVOLVED IN PREPARING INTRAVENOUS ADMIXTURES

The first part of this chapter presents a review of basic mathematics used in performing calculations necessary for preparing I.V. admixtures. This discussion of basic mathematics is not intended to be an exhaustive explanation, but rather a review of material already familiar to the trainee.

FRACTIONS

A fraction is part of a unit quantity—for example, $\frac{1}{2}$. A fraction is composed of two terms, the upper term known as the *numerator* and the lower term the *denominator*. The preferred form of a fraction is to have the denominator larger than the numerator. If the numerator is larger, the denominator can be divided into the numerator to give a whole number and a fraction. For example, $\frac{7}{6}$ is usually expressed as $1\frac{1}{6}$.

Reduction and Enlargement of Fractions A fraction can be reduced to lower terms by dividing the numerator and denominator by the largest multiple common to both. For example, $\frac{9}{12}$ can be reduced to lower terms by dividing the numerator and denominator by 3. Thus, $\frac{9}{12} = \frac{3}{4}$.

A fraction can be raised to higher terms by multiplying the numerator and denominator by the same number. For example, $\frac{2}{3}$ can be raised to higher terms by multiplying the numerator and denominator by 4. Thus, $\frac{2}{3} = \frac{8}{12}$.

The numerator and denominator of a fraction can be multiplied or divided by the same number without changing its value. However, numbers cannot be added to or subtracted from both terms of a fraction and still retain the same value.

Addition and Subtraction of Fractions Before fractions can be added or subtracted, they must have the same denominator. The common denominator is the lowest number into which all denominators can be divided an even number of times. For example, to add $\frac{1}{2}$ and $\frac{2}{3}$, the fractions must have the same denominator, the lowest common denominator being 6. Both $\frac{1}{2}$ and $\frac{2}{3}$ must be raised to higher terms by multiplying by 3 and 2, respectively. Thus, $\frac{1}{2} = \frac{3}{6}$ and $\frac{2}{3} = \frac{4}{6}$. The two fractions are now in a form to be added: $\frac{4}{6} + \frac{3}{6} = \frac{7}{6}$. Similar calculations will shown that $\frac{2}{3} - \frac{1}{2} = \frac{4}{6} - \frac{3}{6} = \frac{1}{6}$.

Multiplication and Division of Fractions To multiply two fractions, multiply the two numerators and the two denominators to get the new numerator and denominator. Thus, to multiply $\frac{1}{6} \times \frac{2}{3}$:

$$\frac{1}{6} \times \frac{2}{3} = \frac{(1 \times 2)}{(6 \times 3)} = \frac{2}{18} = \frac{1}{9}$$

To divide two fractions, invert the divisor (the number that is divided into another number) and then multiply. Thus, to divide $\frac{1}{3}$ by $\frac{1}{4}$:

$$\frac{1}{3} / \frac{1}{4} = \frac{1}{3} \times \frac{4}{1} = \frac{(1 \times 4)}{(3 \times 1)} = \frac{4}{3} = 1\frac{1}{3}$$

Cancellation of Fractions Multiplication of fractions can often be simplified by cancellation—that is, by reducing the numerator of one fraction and the denominator of another. To multiply ⅓ by ⁹⁄₁₆, the following steps could be performed:

$$\frac{1}{3} \times \frac{9}{16} = (1 \times 9)/(3 \times 16) = \frac{9}{48} = \frac{3}{16}$$

However, the calculation could be shortened one step by cancellation:

$$\frac{1}{\underset{1}{\cancel{3}}} \times \frac{\overset{3}{\cancel{9}}}{16} = (1 \times 3) / (1 \times 16) = \frac{3}{16}$$

More than one cancellation can be made when two fractions are multiplied. Thus, to multiply ¾ by ²⁄₉:

$$\frac{\overset{1}{\cancel{3}}}{\underset{2}{\cancel{4}}} \times \frac{\overset{1}{\cancel{2}}}{\underset{3}{\cancel{9}}} = (1 \times 1) / (2 \times 3) = \frac{1}{6}$$

DECIMAL FRACTIONS

Fractions can be converted to decimal fractions by dividing the numerator by the denominator. For example, ⁴⁄₁₀

$$4/10 = 4 \div 10 = 0.4$$

Decimal fractions can be added and subtracted by aligning the decimal points and proceeding as with whole numbers:

0.6	1.2
+0.5	−0.5
1.1	0.7

Multiplication of decimal fractions differs from multiplying whole numbers only in that the decimal point must be properly located. To determine the position of the decimal point, count the total number of digits to the right of the decimal point in each of the numbers that are multiplied. Then point off the same number of places from right to left in the answer. Thus, to multiply 0.43 by 0.29:

```
     .43 (two digits to the right of decimal point)
  X .29 (two digits to the right of decimal point)
    387
   86
  .1247 (four digits to the right of decimal point)
```

If there are fewer digits in the answer than to the right of the decimal point in the numbers multiplied, zeros are added to the extreme left of the answer to provide the proper number of digits. Thus, to multiply 0.43 by 0.21:

```
    .43 (two digits to the right of the decimal)
 X .21 (two digits to the right of the decimal)
     43
    86
 .0903 (need four digits, so add one zero to left)
```

To divide decimal fractions, move the decimal point of both fractions to the same number of decimal places to the right until the divisor is a whole number. When dividing 2.4032 by 0.32, it is easier to determine the position of the decimal point in the answer if the decimal point in each decimal fraction is moved to the right two spaces. The fraction 2.4032/.32 essentially can be multiplied by 100 to yield 240.32/32, which does not alter the value of the fraction, and gives an answer of 7.51.

METRIC SYSTEM OF WEIGHTS AND MEASURES

The system of weights and measures most commonly used in prescriptions today is the metric system. This system is based on the decimal system, in which each unit is related to another by a multiple of 10.

The primary measure of volume is a *liter* (L), which is approximately the volume of one quart. Smaller volumes are measured in *milliliters* (mL or ml), which are one-thousandth of a liter. This volume is also referred to as a *cubic centimeter*, which is seen more commonly in its abbreviated form, cc. The following equations summarize the relationship of volume measurements used in preparing I.V. admixtures:

1 L = 1,000 mL = 1,000 cc
1mL = $\frac{1}{1,000}$ L = 1 cc

The primary measure of weight in the metric system is a *gram*, abbreviated *g*. Amounts of drugs are commonly expressed in grams or milligrams. A *milligram* (*mg*) is one-thousandth of a gram. The relationship between milligrams and grams is the same as that between milliliters and liters. A *microgram* is one-millionth of a gram or one-thousandth of a milligram. A microgram is abbreviated mcg or µg.

1 g = 1,000 mg
1 mg = $\frac{1}{1,000}$ g = 1,000 mcg
1 mcg = $\frac{1}{1,000}$ mg

OTHER SYSTEMS OF WEIGHTS AND MEASURES

Drugs made synthetically are usually very pure and, therefore, measured by weight. The amounts of some drugs from biological sources are expressed in *USP units* or *international units*. Because the potency and purity of drugs from biological sources vary depending on the source, they are measured by units of activity rather than by weight. A unit usually represents an amount equivalent to a certain weight of the pure drug. Drugs commonly measured in units include penicillin, insulin, heparin, and some vitamins.

Another measure of the amount of a drug is the *milliequivalent* (*mEq*). This is the most common way electrolytes such as potassium chloride are expressed. When an electrolyte is dissolved in water, it divides into electrically charged particles (ions). For example, potassium chloride (KCl) splits into a positively charged potassium ion (K^+) and a negatively charged chloride ion (Cl^-). Calcium chloride ($CaCl_2$) disassociates into one calcium ion (Ca^{++}) and two chloride ions (Cl^-). Thus,

$$KCl \iff K^+ + Cl^-$$
$$CaCl_2 \iff Ca^{++} + 2\ Cl^-$$

Note that the positive charges always balance the negative charges. The two-way arrow indicates that the reaction is dynamic, where the ions continuously dissociate and return to salt form of the electrolyte.

Virtually any *cation* (positively charged particle) can combine with any *anion* (negatively charged particle). One milliequivalent of any cation is chemically equivalent to one milliequivalent of any anion. The weight of a chemical has no relation to its chemical activity. For example, 1 mEq of chloride (35 mg) combines with 1 mEq of sodium (23 mg), potassium (39 mg), or calcium (20 mg). This is why electrolytes are expressed in milliequivalents rather than weight. Expressing electrolytes in milliequivalents takes into consideration the number of ions present and their electrical charges, which is a measure of chemical combining ability or chemical activity.

Physicians use the above systems to prescribe a specific amount of drug additive, and all of them will be encountered by admixture personnel.

PERCENTAGE

Fractions with denominators of 100 can be expressed as a percentage; for example, $^3/_{100} = 3\%$, $^1/_{10} = {}^{10}/_{100} = 10\%$, and $^1/_4 = {}^{25}/_{100} = 25\%$. Decimal fractions can be converted to percentage by moving the decimal two places to the right and adding the percent sign. Thus, $0.25 = 25\%$ and $0.10 = 10\%$.

To change percentage to fractions or decimal fractions, the above steps are reversed:

$25\% = {}^{25}/_{100} = {}^1/_4$ $25\% = 0.25$
$10\% = {}^{10}/_{100} = {}^1/_{10}$ $10\% = 0.10$

The strength of many solutions is expressed as a percentage (examples: 5% dextrose injection and 0.9% sodium chloride injection). The percentage strength represents a certain weight, in grams, of a drug in 100 mL of solution. A 5% dextrose injection contains 5 g of dextrose per 100 mL of solution. A 0.9% sodium chloride injection contains 0.9 g of sodium chloride per 100 mL of solution.

PROPORTIONS

Proportions are a means of expressing a fraction in a different form without changing the value. If $^1/_{10}$ is to be converted to hundredths, a proportion can be established to determine how many $^1/_{100}$s equal $^1/_{10}$. If *x* represents the unknown quantity of hundredths, the following expression can be used:

$$^1/_{10} = {}^x/_{100}$$

To solve the proportion, the numerator of one fraction is multiplied by the denominator of the other fraction. The 1 in the left fraction is multiplied by 100 in the right fraction. Then the 10 in the left fraction is multiplied by the x in the right fraction. The results of the cross multiplication are equal, so:

$$10 \times x = 1 \times 100$$

x, the quantity to be determined, is isolated on one side of the equal sign by performing the necessary arithmetic.

	$1/10 = x/100$
(cross-multiplying)	$10 \times x = 1 \times 100$
(multiplying each side)	$10x = 100$
(dividing each side by 10)	$x = 10$
	Thus, $1/10 = 10/100$

The answer may have been obvious without cross-multiplying the fractions, but other proportions may not be as simple. To express $4/25$ in tenths, cross-multiplication is almost necessary.

$4/25 = x/10$

$25 \times x = 4 \times 10$

$25x = 40$

$x = 40/25 = 8/5 = 1.6$

Thus, $4/25 = 1.6/10$

Proportions are used extensively in the preparation of I.V. admixtures. Gentamicin solution is available in 2-mL vials, with each vial containing 80 mg. If a medication order is received for 60 mg of gentamicin in an I.V. solution, a proportion can be set up to determine what volume of gentamicin should be withdrawn from the vial to supply 60 mg.

setting up the proportion:	80 mg/2 mL = 60 mg/x
cross-multiplying:	80 mg $\times$ x = 60 mg $\times$ 2 mL
multiplying each side:	80 mg x = 120 mg mL
canceling *mg* each side:	$80x = 120$ mL
dividing each side by 80:	$x = 1.5$ mL

Thus, a volume of 1.5 mL of solution must be withdrawn from the vial to supply 60 mg of gentamicin. It is essential to include units of measure in all calculations to assure the accuracy of the answer.

ALLIGATION

If a certain percentage strength of a solution is needed but it is not available, it can be made by combining a stronger solution with a weaker one to provide the desired strength. *Alligation* is the process of determining the proportion of each component to use in preparing a solution of a specific strength. The scheme used to solve this type of problem is as follows:

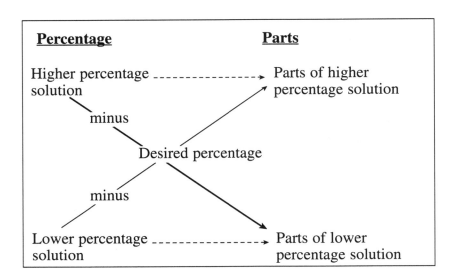

The percentages of the components to be used in compounding the final product are written on the left corners of the rectangle. The final percentage desired is written in the center.

The relative parts required are calculated and written on the right corners of the rectangle. The desired percentage is subtracted from the higher percentage to give the parts of the lower percentage solution needed, which is written in the lower right corner. The lower percentage is subtracted from the desired percentage to give the parts of the higher percentage solution needed, which is written in the upper right corner.

Once the proportional parts have been determined, the quantities of each component needed for a certain total quantity can be determined by proportion.

An example may illustrate the preceding explanation of alligation. A prescription calls for 1,000 mL of a parenteral nutrition solution with 20% dextrose. The most concentrated solution of dextrose immediately available is 50%. What volume of 50% dextrose must be used to prepare a final dextrose concentration of 20%?

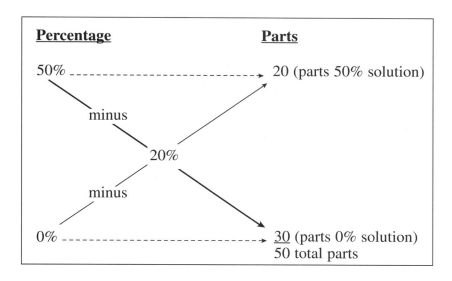

Twenty parts of 50% dextrose can be mixed with 30 parts of 0% dextrose solution (amino acids and sterile water) to give a final concentration of 20% dextrose. The quantity of each component is established by solving a proportion.

$$\frac{\text{parts 50\% dextrose solution}}{\text{total parts}} = \frac{\text{volume 50\% dextrose solution}}{\text{total volume}}$$

All quantities are known in the above proportion except the volume of 50% dextrose solution required, so let that quantity equal x.

20 parts/50 parts = x/1,000 mL
50 parts X x = 20 parts X 1000 mL
50 x parts = 20,000 mL parts
50x = 20,000 mL
x = 20,000 mL/50 = 400 mL

Since the 50% dextrose solution accounts for 400 mL of the final volume, the solution with 0% dextrose must have a volume of 600 mL. Thus,

400 mL of 50% dextrose solution
+ 600 mL of 0% dextrose solution
1,000 mL of 20% dextrose solution

The basic mathematical methods necessary to work most problems associated with preparing I.V. admixtures have been presented. It is beneficial if the reasonableness of all answers is checked by estimating the answer prior to the actual calculation. Ideally, all calculations should be checked by a pharmacist before an admixture is prepared, but they must be checked before an admixture is dispensed.

PRACTICE PROBLEMS

The rest of this chapter is devoted to practice problems and their solutions. For maximum benefit, the problems should be attempted before the answers are known.

Problem 1 A prescription requires 7,500 units(U) of heparin. Heparin vials containing 1,000 U per milliliter are available in the pharmacy. What volume of heparin injection should be added to the I.V. solution to provide 7,500 U?

Solution:

$1,000$ U/mL $= 7,500$ U/x

$1,000$ U X $x = 7,500$ U X mL

1000 U $x = 7500$ U mL

$1,000x = 7,500$ mL

$x = 7,500/1,000$ mL

$x = 7.5$ mL

Thus, 7.5 mL of heparin (1,000 U/mL) should be added to provide the 7,500-U dose.

Problem 2 A 200-mg dose of cimetidine is prescribed. It is available in the pharmacy in 300 mg/2 mL vials. What volume should be withdrawn from the vial to provide a 200-mg dose?

Solution:

300 mg/2 mL $= 200$ mg/x

300 mg X $x = 2$ mL X 200 mg

300 mg $x = 400$ mL mg

300 $x = 400$ mL

$x = 400/300$ mL

$x = 1.33$ mL

Thus, 1.33 mL should be withdrawn to provide a 200-mg dose of cimetidine.

Problem 3 A prescription for 1 L of an admixture to be infused over a period of eight hours is received. If the administration set delivers 10 drops (gtt) per milliliter, what infusion rate, in drops per minute, should appear on the label of the admixture?

Solution:

converting L to mL:

$\qquad$ 1 L/8 hr $= 1,000$ mL/8 hr $= 125$ mL/hr

converting hours to minutes:

$\qquad$ 125 mL/hr $= 125$ mL/60 min $= 2.1$ mL/min

converting mL to drops:

$\qquad$ 2.1 mL/min $= 21$ gtt/min

Thus, the admixture should be infused at a rate of 21 gtt/min to deliver 1 L over a period of eight hours.

Problem 4 Ceftriaxone is available in a 10-g bulk pharmacy container, which is convenient for mass reconstitution and preparation of several admixtures at one time. (See chapter 9.) Rather than reconstituting individual 500-mg or 1-g vials, one 10-g bulk vial can be reconstituted to make the compounding process more efficient.

The package insert states that 95 mL can be added to the 10-g bulk pharmacy container to give a final concentration of 100 mg/mL. What volume of diluent should be added to provide a final concentration of 200 mg/mL?

Solution:

If the final concentration is 100 mg/mL, the final volume must be 100 mL (i.e., 10 g / 100 mg/mL) to provide a total of 10 g. Since only 95 mL of diluent is added and the final volume is 100 mL, the ceftriaxone powder must account for the equivalent of 5 mL of volume. Thus,

$$\begin{array}{r} 95 \text{ mL suitable diluent} \\ + \quad 5 \text{ mL (equivalent) ceftriaxone powder} \\ \hline 100 \text{ mL ceftriaxone solution (100 mg/mL)} \end{array}$$

If the final concentration desired is 200 mg/mL, a final volume of 50 mL will account for all of the ceftriaxone solution. However, the ceftriaxone powder still occupies the same volume, inasmuch as no change has been made in the amount to be reconstituted. Thus,

$$\begin{array}{r} x \text{ mL suitable diluent} \\ + \quad 5 \text{ mL (equivalent) ceftriaxone powder} \\ \hline 50 \text{ mL ceftriaxone solution (200 mg/mL)} \end{array}$$

Then x = 50 mL - 5 mL = 45 mL. Thus, add 45 mL of sterile water for injection to provide a final concentration of 200 mg/mL.

Problem 5 A prescription is received for drug additives in 500 mL of 8% dextrose injection. No solution of 8% dextrose injection is available, but 500-mL bags of 5%, 10%, 20%, and 50% dextrose injection are available. How can 8% dextrose injection be prepared?

Solution:

Alligation can be used to solve this problem by using 5% and 10% dextrose injections, although any two dextrose solutions could be used if one concentration is greater than 8% and one is less than 8%.

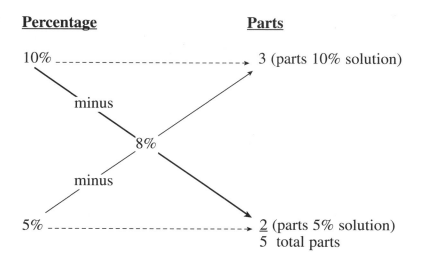

A proportion can be established to determine the unknown quantity. The total volume of 500 mL represents a total of 5 parts, 3 parts of which must be 10% dextrose injection. Here x represents the unknown volume of 10% dextrose solution to be added.

$$\frac{\text{parts 10\% dextrose}}{\text{total parts}} = \frac{\text{volume 10\% dextrose}}{\text{total volume}}$$

3 parts/5 parts = x/500 mL
5 parts × x = 3 parts × 500 mL
5 parts x = 1,500 parts mL
5x = 1,500 mL
x = 300 mL

Thus, 300 mL of 10% dextrose injection should be added to 200 mL of 5% dextrose injection to provide 500 mL of 8% dextrose injection.

Problem 6 A prescription is received for 1L of a parenteral nutrition solution with a final concentration of 15% dextrose. The physician specifies that 500 mL is to be an amino acid solution. The pharmacy has 50% dextrose injection in 500-mL bags. How would this prescription be prepared?

Solution:

First calculate the volume of 50% dextrose injection needed to give the final solution of 1,000 mL a concentration of 15% dextrose.

15% = 15 g/100 mL = 150 g/1000 mL

The 150 g of dextrose must be provided from the 50% dextrose solution, so it must be determined what volume of 50% dextrose solution is needed.

50% = 50 g/100 mL = 150 g/300 mL

Thus, to adjust the final concentration to 15%, 300 mL of 50% dextrose injection is added to 500 mL of the amino acid solution. Then 200 mL of sterile water for injection is added to provide a total volume of 1,000 mL.

Problem 7 Tobramycin may be administered to neonates at a dose of up to 4 mg/kg/day in two equal doses every 12 hours. One kilogram (kg) = 1,000 g = approximately 2.2 lb. In addition to an adult-size multiple dose vial, tobramycin is available in a pediatric vial with a concentration of 20 mg/2 mL. If the neonate weighs 4.0 lb, what volume of tobramycin should be withdrawn for the dose described above?

Solution:

Since the dose of 4 mg/kg/day is in two equally divided doses, each dose would be 2 mg/kg.

The patient weighs 4.0 lb
thus, (4 lb) × (1 kg/2.2 lb) = 1.82 kg

Each dose is (2 mg/kg) × (1.82 kg) = 3.64 mg

The injection is available as 20 mg/2 mL

then 3.64 mg/x = 20 mg/2 mL

20 mg × x = 3.64 mg × 2 mL

20 mg x = 7.28 mg mL

20x = 7.28 mL

x = 0.36 mL

Thus, 0.36 mL of the pediatric strength (20 mg/2 mL) is required for the neonatal dose. A syringe that has a long, slender barrel and a 1-mL capacity is recommended. Extra care should be taken in calculating pediatric and neonatal doses. Doses that are very small amounts should also be double-checked.

Problem 8 As with many drugs, the dose of dobutamine is determined by the size of the patient. The patient weighs 70 kg. The physician prescribes 250 mg/L of dobutamine and wants it to be administered at a rate of 5 mcg/kg/min. 1 mcg = $^1/_{1,000}$ mg. How fast should the solution be administered, in milligrams per hour, to deliver the prescribed dose?

Solution:

First, calculating the dose:

5 mcg/kg/min × 70 kg = 350 mcg/min = 21,000 mcg/hr

Next, calculating the solution strength:

250 mg/1,000 mL = 250,000 mcg/1,000 mL = 250 mcg/mL

Converting the dose from mcg to mL:

21,000 mcg/hr ÷ 250 mcg/mL = 84 mL/hr

CHAPTER 8
FACILITIES, EQUIPMENT, AND SUPPLIES

FACILITIES LAYOUT

A centralized pharmacy admixture service can be operated from a reasonably small area if it is well planned. The centralized admixture area should have limited access and be separated from other pharmacy operations. It may be a separate room, in which case it should be immediately adjacent to the dispensing and order-processing areas of the pharmacy to facilitate communication. Alternatively, the admixture preparation area may be located in a low-traffic area within the pharmacy.

The I.V. admixture area should be clean and well lighted. Sterile products are prepared in laminar air flow hoods (discussed later in this chapter). Other equipment may include a refrigerator, a freezer, and supply carts. A sink for handwashing should be close by. The facility should be laid out to minimize the potential for airborne contamination to come in contact with the products being prepared. Therefore, materials that generate large amounts of particles (e.g., cardboard boxes) should not be permitted in the area. The I.V. admixture area, including the floor, walls, and equipment, should also be cleaned and disinfected regularly.

The layout should also be designed for the efficient flow of orders. As orders are processed, they should pass from one area to an immediately adjacent area. For example, the most frequently used drugs and solutions should be conveniently accessible from the admixture assembly counter so that several orders can be efficiently set up at one time. Once the components of the admixture orders have been assembled on the counter, one order at a time can be taken into the laminar flow hood, compounded, and placed on the admixture checking counter with very little lost motion. An example of an efficiently designed floor plan is shown in figure 8.1.

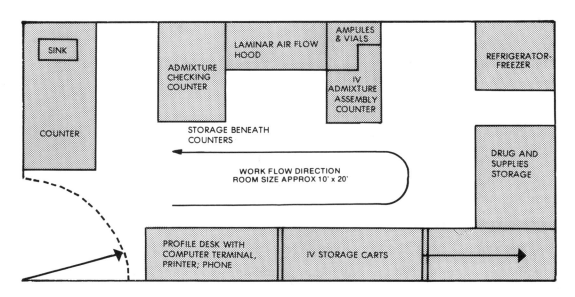

FIGURE 8.1. LAYOUT OF ADMIXTURE PREPARATION AREA

Although the layout of the admixture preparation area depends on the volume of orders processed, the basic elements for designing the area are the same. For example, more sophisticated operations may include a separate support area, or anteroom, adjacent to the actual compounding area. Functions such as entering orders, generating labels, and gathering supplies are performed in the anteroom, which acts as a buffer area that reduces the particle burden in the compounding room. Some facilities have incorporated positive air pressure and special filters into the air-conditioning systems to reduce particulate contamination. Figure 8.2 shows a layout that incorporates a separate anteroom and gowning area.

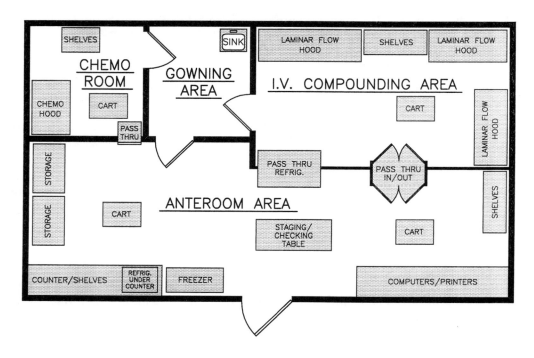

FIGURE 8.2. LAYOUT OF ADMIXTURE PREPARATION AREA WITH ANTEROOM

EQUIPMENT

Computers Most hospital pharmacies now use computers to carry out a variety of tasks related to the I.V. admixture service. Common tasks include:

- Generating labels
- Maintaining a profile of current orders
- Screening for incompatibilities and duplicate orders
- Inquiring into an on-line patient medical record to access information such as diagnosis and laboratory test results
- Generating patient charges
- Maintaining work-load and product-usage records
- Generating mass-production or batch-compounding worksheets
- Updating drug costs

Although entering an order into a computer (figure 8.3) takes a little longer than typing a single label on a typewriter, the investment of time continues to produce benefits for as long as the order is active. Once the order is entered into the computer, labels can be requested for certain time intervals to correspond with major admixture compounding times and can be printed by patient, nursing unit, drug, time, etc., to help in the sorting process. Most of the other tasks listed above occur automatically as a by-product of the order entry process.

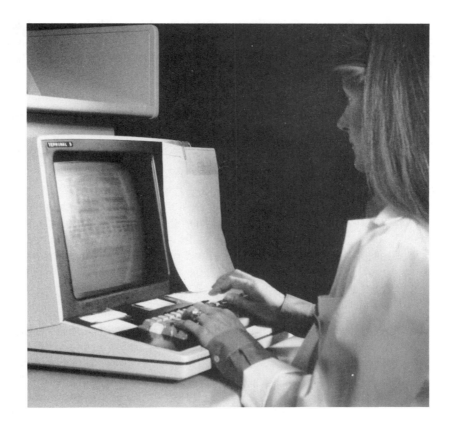

FIGURE 8.3. COMPUTER FOR PHARMACY APPLICATIONS

Orders can be entered into the computer by using a light pen or a "mouse" to select from a menu of options displayed on the screen or by using a keyboard to type in free text or to select from various options. Some pharmacies use bar codes to enter medication order data into computers by scanning common standardized order sets. Voice recognition technology, which actually allows users to talk to the computer to enter orders, is an exciting future capability for improving efficiency.

Three types of computers are commonly used in hospital pharmacies:

- *A pharmacy system* that runs on the organization's mainframe computer. Terminals and printers in the pharmacy, as well as in other departments, are linked directly to the mainframe computer to allow access to information across departments.

- *A stand-alone system* that runs on a minicomputer dedicated to the pharmacy. This type of system may or may not be linked to the hospital's mainframe computer, although it is generally interfaced for admission/discharge/transfer data and billing functions.

- *A personal computer* that is useful in maintaining profiles of active orders and in generating labels if a larger computer system is not feasible.

The health care system of the future will create a much greater need to access and share patient information across departments and organizations. Pharmacy data regarding medications must be shared with the clinical laboratories and other departments. Likewise, the pharmacy will need to have access to laboratory test results that may show electrolyte levels or culture and sensitivity tests to antibiotics. A clinical database that includes all information in the patient record will become increasingly important as a means of analyzing costs and developing a comprehensive, on-line medical record. Not only is this type of electronic medical record needed for sharing data within the hospital, but it will also need to be accessible to other health care organizations such as physicians' offices, ambulatory care clinics, long-term care facilities, hospice programs, home care agencies, and outpatient pharmacies that are partners within the same managed care system. Clearly, time is running out for the pharmacy that operates as an independent department with no computer or with a stand-alone computer not closely integrated with the health system mainframe computer.

Laminar Flow Hoods Laminar flow hoods are designed to reduce the risk of airborne contamination during the preparation of I.V. admixtures by providing an ultraclean environment. Thus, a more suitable preparation area than that provided in a patient care area is another advantage of an admixture program in the pharmacy.

The most important part of a laminar flow hood is a high-efficiency, bacteria-retentive filter, commonly called a HEPA (High-Efficiency Particulate Air) filter. As seen in figure 8.4, room air is taken into the unit and passed through a prefilter to remove relatively large contaminants such as dust and lint. The air is then compressed and channeled up behind and through the high-efficiency filter, where nearly all bacteria are removed. The purified air then flows out over the entire work surface in parallel lines at a uniform velocity (i.e., _laminar flow_).

A laminar flow hood has three basic functions. The first is to provide clean air in the working area. This is accomplished by passing room air through a bacteria-retentive filter to provide a continuous flow of clean air in the work area. Second, the constant flow of air out of the laminar flow hood prevents room air from entering the work area. Last, the air flowing out suspends and removes contaminants introduced into the work area by material (e.g., I.V. solution containers) or personnel. Thus, a laminar flow hood provides an environment virtually free of airborne contaminants in which procedures can be safely performed.

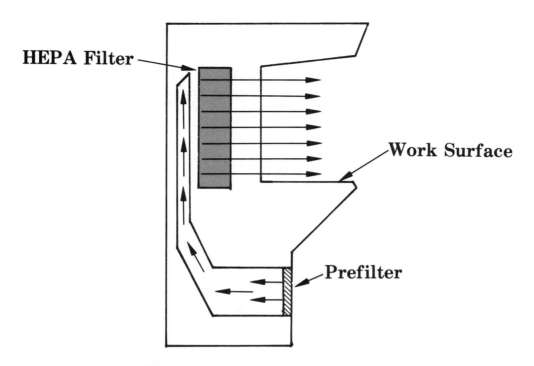

FIGURE 8.4. LAMINAR FLOW HOOD, SIDE VIEW

Laminar flow hoods may be used in the pharmacy to perform the following procedures:

- Preparation of I.V. admixtures
- Preparation of ophthalmic solutions
- Reconstitution of powdered drugs
- Filling unit dose syringes
- Preparation of miscellaneous sterile products

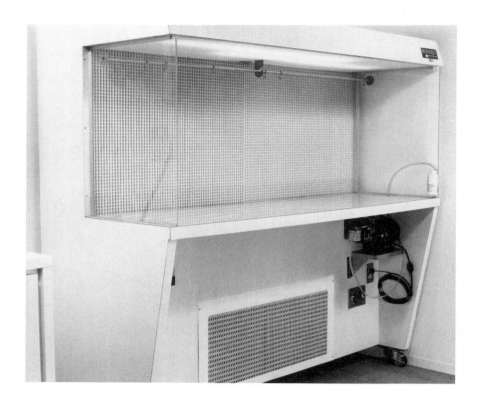

FIGURE 8.5. CONSOLE LAMINAR FLOW HOOD

Laminar flow units commonly used in admixture programs are the bench and the console models. The console model, shown in figure 8.5, sits on the floor and is available in several different sizes, most commonly ranging from 3 ft to 6 ft in length. As figure 8.4 shows, room air is taken in at the bottom of the unit and channeled upward, through the bacteria-retentive filter, and out horizontally across the work surface in a laminar flow fashion.

The bench (counter top) model, as shown in figure 8.6, is also available in several different sizes. Because the space under the laminar flow hood can be used for storage, the unit provides a clean work area with minimum use of floor space. Room air enters at the top of the unit and is channeled downward, through the bacteria-retentive filter, and out horizontally across the work surface.

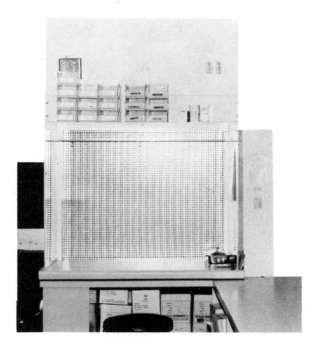

FIGURE 8.6. BENCH LAMINAR FLOW HOOD

Both the console and bench models are available with vertical rather than horizontal air flow. With vertical flow, room air enters at the top of the unit and is channeled through the bacteria-retentive filter, which forms the ceiling of the unit, and down vertically across the work surface. Although the horizontal- and vertical-flow units are equally effective, the horizontal flow is more commonly used in admixture programs. (See chapter 11 for discussion of special hoods for compounding chemotherapy solutions.)

Laminar air flow hoods are usually kept running continuously. If the hood is turned off, it should be run for at least 30 minutes before use to replace with clean, filtered air the room air that has entered the hood work area while the hood has been off.

Laminar flow hoods should be inspected and certified every six months to assure that the HEPA filter is intact, i.e., that it has no holes and is not clogged. The prefilters in the hoods should be changed monthly.

SUPPLIES

Needles Basically, a needle consists of two parts—the shaft and the hub. As shown in figure 8.7, the *shaft* is the long, slender stem of the needle that is *beveled* (i.e., the diagonal cut of the shaft) at one end to form a point. The hollow bore of the needle shaft is known as the *lumen*. At the other end of the needle is the *hub*, to which a syringe can be attached.

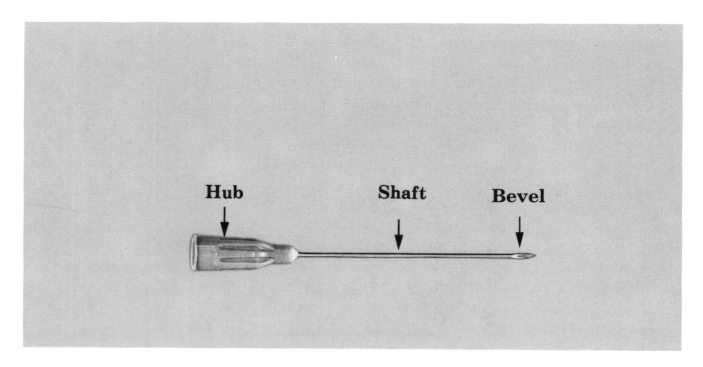

FIGURE 8.7. PARTS OF A NEEDLE

Needle size is designated by length and gauge. The length of a needle is measured in inches from the juncture of the hub and the shaft to the tip of the point. Needle lengths range from ⅜ in. to 3½ in. or longer. The *gauge* of a needle, used to designate the size of the lumen, ranges from 27, the finest, to 13, the largest. The finer the needle, the higher the gauge number. In some disposable needles, the gauge is designated by the color of the hub in order to facilitate recognition. One factor in choosing a needle size is the thickness (*viscosity*) of the injectable solution. Fine needles with a relatively small lumen may be acceptable for most solutions, but needles with a larger lumen (and a smaller gauge number) may be needed for viscous solutions. Another factor in selecting the proper needle is the nature of the rubber closure to be penetrated. Fine needles with a smaller lumen may be preferred for rubber closures that *core* easily (i.e., small particles of rubber are broken away and carried into the drug solution when the needle penetrates the rubber closure).

Disposable needles should always be used when preparing admixtures, as they are presterilized and individually wrapped to maintain sterility.

Syringes The two basic parts of a syringe are the barrel and the plunger (figure 8.8). The *barrel* is a tube that is open at one end and tapers into a hollow tip at the other end. The open end is extended radially outward to form a rim, or *flange*, to prevent the barrel from slipping through the fingers during manipulation.

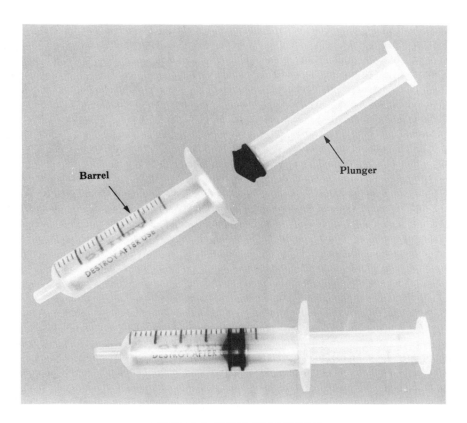

FIGURE 8.8. PARTS OF A SYRINGE

The *plunger* is a piston-type rod with a slightly cone-shaped tip that passes inside the barrel of the syringe. The other end of the plunger is shaped into a flat knob for easy manipulation. The plunger must be able to move freely throughout the barrel, yet its surface must be so close to the barrel that the fluid cannot pass between them, even when under considerable pressure.

The tip of the syringe provides the point of attachment for a needle. The tip may be tapered to allow the needle hub to be slipped over it and held on by friction. When this method is used, the needle is reasonably secure, but it may slip off if not properly attached or if considerable pressure is used to inject the solution. Locking devices have been developed to secure the needle more firmly on the tip of the syringe; one such device has the trade name Luer-Lok. These devices incorporate a collar with a circular internal groove into which the needle hub is inserted. A half-turn locks the needle in place. This method is especially valuable when pressure is required.

The volume of solution inside a syringe is indicated by graduation lines on the barrel. Accurate readings are more easily made if the color of the tip of the plunger is different from that of the syringe itself. Common disposable syringes have a capacity of 1-60 mL. Graduation lines may be in milliliters or fractions of a milliliter, depending on the capacity of the syringe, i.e., the larger the capacity, the larger the interval between graduation lines. Special-purpose syringes, such as insulin syringes, have graduation lines in both milliliters and insulin units to reflect their intended use (figure 8.9).

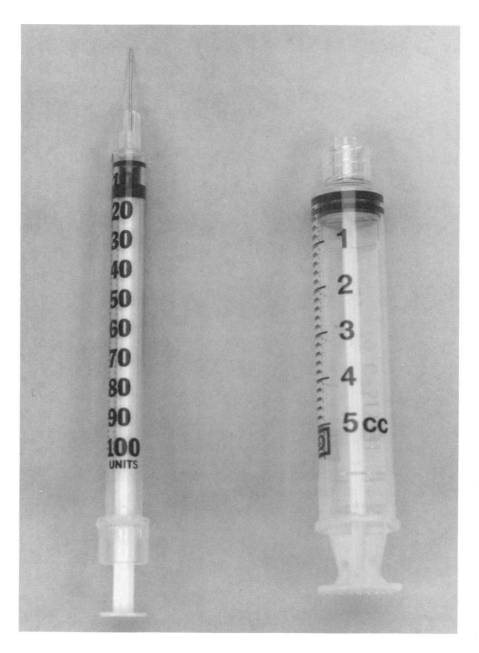

FIGURE 8.9. COMPARISON OF INSULIN AND REGULAR SYRINGES

In the selection of an appropriate syringe, as a general rule the capacity of the syringe should be the next size larger than the volume to be measured. For example, a 3-mL syringe should be selected to measure a 2.3-mL dose, or a 5-mL syringe to measure a 3.8-mL dose. In this way, the graduation marks on the syringe will be in the smallest possible increments for the dose measured. Syringes should not be filled to capacity, however, because the plunger can be easily dislodged. As discussed in chapter 11, to avoid this problem, it is recommended that syringes containing chemotherapy drugs not be filled more than three-quarters of capacity.

Sterile disposable syringes are discarded after one use and have the same advantages as disposable needles. Although syringes made of either plastic or disposable glass are available, plastic is usually used because of its lower cost, unless a drug is incompatible with the plastic.

Some pharmaceutical manufacturers supply common doses of frequently used or emergency-use drugs in prefilled syringes. Prefilled syringes eliminate the need to measure doses, thus saving valuable time in compounding admixtures. Examples of prefilled syringes are shown in figure 8.10.

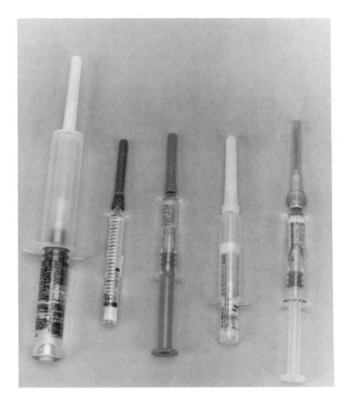

FIGURE 8.10. PREFILLED SYRINGES

Sometimes it may be desirable to provide a drug additive or other sterile product to the patient care area in a predrawn syringe rather than a minibag. Appropriate occasions may include administration of an antibiotic through a volume control chamber to a pediatric patient or a patient with a severe fluid restriction, or I.V. push administration of an anesthesia drug in surgery. In order to maintain the sterility of the drug drawn into a syringe, the tip of the syringe must be sealed with a sterile cap or the needle must be reattached. A sterile syringe cap is shown in figure 8.11.

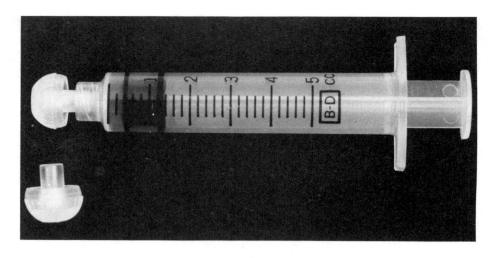

FIGURE 8.11. SYRINGE CAPS

SOLUTION CONTAINERS

I.V. solution containers are of two basic types: plastic bags and glass bottles. Containers made by the three manufacturers of I.V. solutions may vary somewhat, but they all have the same essential features.

Plastic Bags The most common I.V. administration system is the plastic bag system, as shown in figure 8.12.

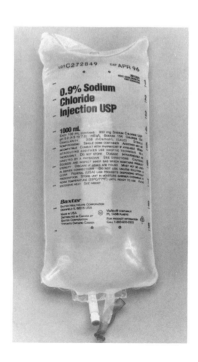

FIGURE 8.12. PLASTIC I.V. BAG

Plastic bags are available in different sizes, with 50, 100, 250, 500, and 1,000 mL being the most common. Special bags for compounding parenteral nutrition are available in 2,000- and 3,000-mL sizes. At the top of the bag is a flat plastic extension with a hole to allow it to be hung on an administration pole. At the other end of the bag are two ports of about the same length. One port, the administration set port, has a blue plastic cover similar to that on the end of an administration set. The plastic cover, which serves to maintain the sterility of the administration set port, is easily removed. Once the plastic cover is pulled off, the sterile port for the administration set is exposed. Solution will not drip from the plastic bag at this point because of a plastic diaphragm about ½ in. inside the port. The spike of the administration set is inserted into the port, puncturing the inner diaphragm to allow the solution to flow from the flexible plastic bag into the administration set. Once punctured, the inner diaphragm is not resealable.

The other port, the medication port, is covered by a protective rubber tip. Medication is added to the solution through this medication port by means of a needle and syringe. The rubber tip is self-sealing, thus preventing solution from leaking when the tip is punctured by the needle. Approximately ½ in. inside this port is a plastic diaphragm that must be punctured to enter the bag. The inner diaphragm is not self-sealing when punctured by a needle, so the rubber tip must remain in place.

Graduation marks to indicate the volume of solution infused are located on both sides of the front of some plastic bags at 25-100 mL intervals, depending on their capacity.

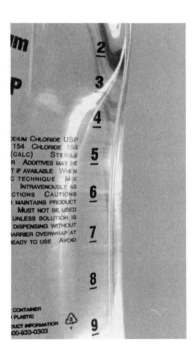

FIGURE 8.13. GRADUATION MARKS ON PLASTIC I.V. BAG

Labeling on plastic bags, printed on one side, contains the usual descriptive and quality control information for all drugs as described in chapter 3. Some pharmacists prefer to affix the admixture label on the nonprinted side of the bag to avoid obscuring the printed labeling. Others prefer to affix the admixture label on the printed side of the bag, beneath the solution name and offset slightly to one side so that the graduation marks near the side can still be read. The latter procedure has the advantage of providing a convenient cross-check between the actual solution and that appearing on the admixture label. The label is attached in an upright position to enable easy reading when the plastic bag is hung for administration (figure 8.14).

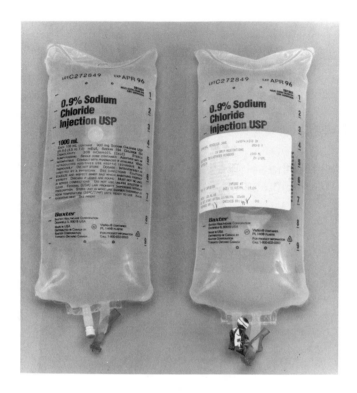

FIGURE 8.14. PLASTIC BAG SHOWING MANUFACTURER'S LABELING AND ADMIXTURE LABEL

Some I.V. solutions, such as 5% dextrose injection and 0.9% sodium chloride injection, are available in minibags or piggyback bags. These bags typically hold 50 mL or 100 mL of solution and are used to administer drugs, such as antibiotics, intermittently rather than continuously (see figure 8.15).

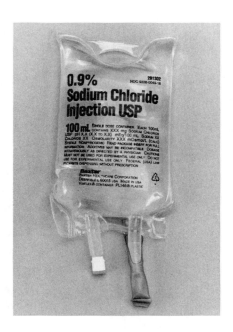

FIGURE 8.15. MINIBAG

The plastic bag system is completely closed to outside air. It does not depend on outside air to displace the solution as it leaves the bag. The bag collapses as the solution is administered, so a vacuum is not created inside.

Tamperproof plastic caps or paper seals, which fit over the medication port, are available for use with the plastic bag system. When the cap or seal is in place, it signifies that a medication has been added to the solution and that the admixture has not been tampered with since being dispensed from the pharmacy (see figure 8.16).

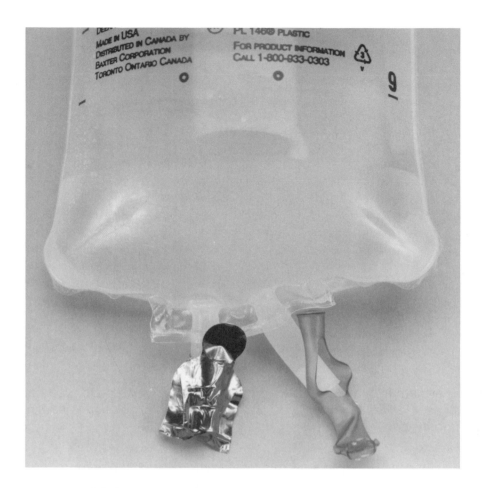

FIGURE 8.16. TAMPERPROOF CLOSURE FOR PLASTIC I.V. BAG

Glass Bottles Because of the advantages afforded by plastic I.V. bags (i.e., it is a system not dependent on outside air and thus referred to as a closed system; they do not break; they weigh less; they take up less storage space; they take up much less disposal space), glass I.V. solution bottles are used relatively infrequently. Their major advantage is in administering drugs that are incompatible with plastic.

Glass I.V. bottles are packaged under a vacuum and sealed by a rubber closure held in place by an aluminum band. For the solution to flow from the glass bottles, the vacuum must be released and the solution displaced by air as it is administered.

The closure of the glass I.V. bottle is solid rubber. Filtered air enters the bottle through an airway that is an integral part of the administration set spike. (This is sometimes referred to as a vented spike or vented set.)

The glass solution bottles described above can be sealed with a tamperproof closure (figure 8.17) after the admixture is prepared. Although tamperproof closures differ in appearance, depending on the manufacturer, they function in the same manner. Because it must be torn to be removed, a tamperproof closure still intact provides assurance that an admixture has not been altered since it was prepared in the pharmacy.

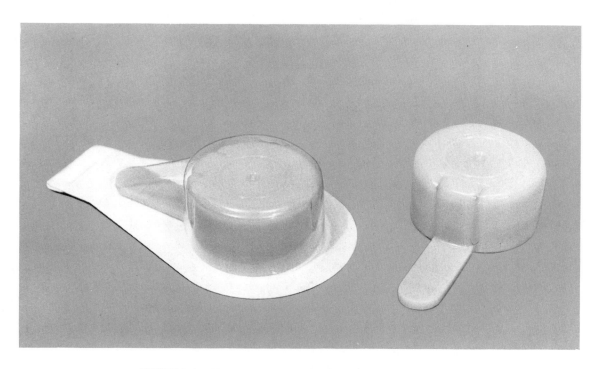

FIGURE 8.17. TAMPERPROOF CLOSURE FOR GLASS I.V. BOTTLE

Along the side of the bottle, molded graduation marks show the solution volume in both the upright and inverted position (figure 8.18). Graduation marks are usually spaced every 20-50 mL to facilitate reading. The solution bottle is hung in an inverted position by an aluminum or plastic band located at the bottom of the bottle.

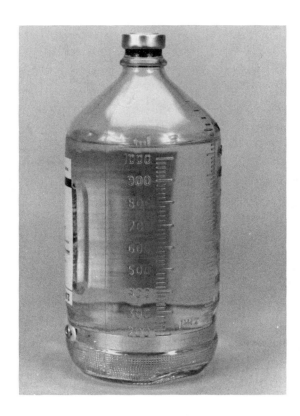

FIGURE 8.18. GLASS I.V. BOTTLE

The admixture label should be affixed over the manufacturer's label in an inverted position just below the manufacturer's inverted identification. Positioning the label in this manner makes it easier to read the admixture label when the solution is administered and also provides a means to make sure that the solution used in preparing the admixture is the same as that shown on the label.

Some I.V. solutions, such as 5% dextrose injection and 0.9% sodium chloride injection, are also available in partially filled solution bottles known as minibottles or piggyback bottles. Minibottles contain 50 mL or 100 mL of solution in a 250-mL capacity bottle and, like piggyback bags, are used to administer drugs intermittently.

FILTERS

A *filter* is a device through which a solution is passed to remove particles. A filter may be used during compounding as an attachment on the end of a syringe or as an integral part of the hub of the needle. Alternatively, filters may be used in conjunction with an administration set to clarify solutions immediately before they are infused into the patient. These filters may be built into the set or may be attached to the end of the set.

In general, filters may be divided into two broad groups: depth filters and membrane filters. Depth filters trap particles by passing the solution through tortuous channels, thereby clarifying the solution. A depth filter, made of stainless steel, is shown in figure 8.19. A membrane filter, which looks like paper, consists of meshwork of millions of microcapillary pores of uniform size. These filters are made in the form of films 1-200 microns thick (a *micron* is about 4/100,000 of an inch) and trap particles larger than the size of the pores. A membrane filter attached to a needle and syringe is shown in figure 8.20.

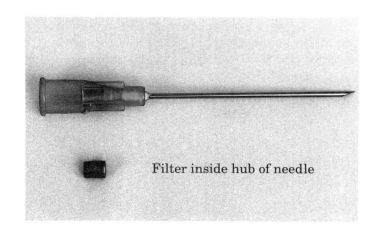

Filter inside hub of needle

FIGURE 8.19. DEPTH FILTER

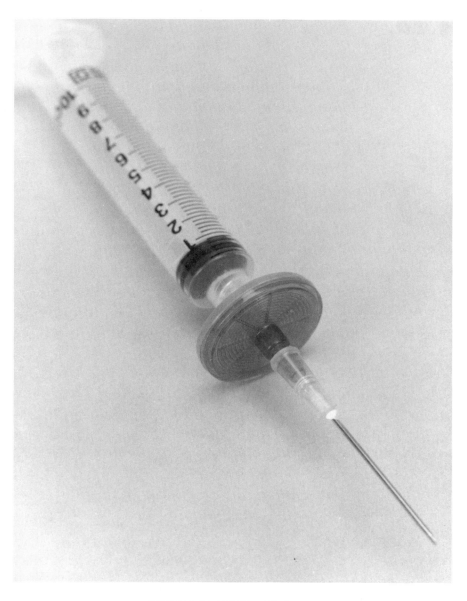

FIGURE 8.20. MEMBRANE FILTER

Both the depth filter and the membrane filter are available in a wide range of pore sizes. A 0.22-micron pore size is considered to be a sterilizing filter capable of removing all microorganisms. Other sizes commonly used in the pharmacy and suitable for clarifying solutions have a porosity of 0.45, 1, 5, or 10 microns.

CHAPTER 9

TECHNIQUES USED IN PREPARING INTRAVENOUS ADMIXTURES

ASEPTIC TECHNIQUE

Aseptic technique refers to carrying out a procedure under controlled conditions in a manner that minimizes the chance of contamination caused by the introduction of microorganisms. Because contaminants may be introduced from the environment, equipment and supplies, or personnel, it is essential to control these different sources of contamination at the time aseptic technique is carried out.

__Environment__ Environmental control of the air is of concern because room air may be highly contaminated. A laminar flow hood effectively provides high-quality air in the work area for performing aseptic techniques.

__Equipment and Supplies__ All objects that come in contact with the drug additive or I.V. solution must be sterile, or contamination will result. Many of the hazards associated with contamination are eliminated with the use of disposable supplies such as needles and syringes.

__Personnel__ Touch contamination by the person performing a procedure is the most frequent cause of contamination, occurring when proper control over manipulations is not maintained. Good technique in the preparation of I.V. admixtures is critical to producing a sterile product. Handwashing and proper attire are important aspects of aseptic technique designed to control touch contamination.

Following is a suggested handwashing procedure for all I.V. admixture personnel:

1. Remove any hand jewelry, such as rings or watches.
2. Stand far enough away from the sink so that clothing does not come in contact with it.
3. Turn on the water and wet hands and forearms thoroughly. Keep hands pointed downward.
4. Scrub hands vigorously with an antibacterial soap.
5. Work soap under the fingernails by rubbing them against the palm of the other hand.
6. Interlace the fingers and scrub the spaces between the fingers.
7. Wash wrists and arms up to the elbows.
8. Thoroughly rinse the soap from hands and arms.
9. Dry hands and forearms thoroughly using a nonshedding paper towel. (Water left on the skin provides a medium for bacterial growth.)
10. Use a dry paper towel to turn off the water faucet.
11. After hands are washed, avoid touching clothes, face, hair, or any other potentially contaminated object in the area.

A document produced by the American Society of Health-System Pharmacists, *ASHP Technical Assistance Bulletin on Quality Assurance for Pharmacy-Prepared Sterile Products* (Am J Hosp Pharm 1993; 50:2386-98), recommends that the following apparel be worn by personnel during aseptic preparation procedures involving the lowest risk level (higher risk level recommendations are discussed in chapter 13):

- Clean garments or clothing covers that generate low amounts of particles in the controlled area
- Head and facial hair covers
- Mask

The danger in breaking aseptic technique is readily apparent. Not only are patients receiving I.V. admixtures the most critical patients in the hospital, but the I.V. route is the most dangerous route of administration. Because all natural barriers are bypassed when a drug is administered directly into the vein, administration of a contaminated solution can have very serious consequences. Therefore, every precaution must be taken to exercise good aseptic technique in order to avoid contaminating the admixture.

WORKING IN A LAMINAR FLOW HOOD

Because laminar flow air begins to mix with outside air near the edge of the hood, all work should be performed at least 6 in. inside the hood to derive the benefits of the laminar air flow. Technicians should not become so engrossed in their work that they forget this basic rule and perform the work at the edge or even outside the hood.

A direct, open path must be maintained between the filter and the area inside the hood where manipulations are performed. Air downstream from nonsterile objects, such as solution containers or the operator's hands, becomes contaminated from particles blown off these objects. Large objects such as solution containers should not be placed at the back of the work area next to the filter. Not only do these objects contaminate everything downstream, but they also disrupt the laminar flow pattern of the air.

Before and after preparing a series of admixtures, or any time something is spilled, the work surface of the laminar flow hood should be cleaned with 70% isopropyl alcohol or other suitable germicide. A long, side-to-side motion should be used, starting at the back and working forward. The acrylic plastic sides of a laminar flow hood also need routine cleaning. Soap and water are recommended for cleaning acrylic plastic because alcohol may cause a hazy appearance to develop over time.

MEASURING DRUGS WITH A SYRINGE

A needle and syringe can be used to add most drugs to an I.V. solution. This method of adding drug additives can be used for powdered as well as liquid drugs. Disposable needles and syringes are used for this transfer, and both are supplied sterile in individual packages. The appropriate size syringe is selected based on the volume of solution to be measured and the graduation marks on the syringe. The smallest size syringe should be selected, but it should not be filled to capacity. Selecting the smallest size syringe allows the volume to measured most accurately because of the smaller interval between graduation marks. As a general rule, syringes should not be filled to capacity because the plunger can be dislodged too easily.

The needle is attached to the syringe by the following procedure:

1. Remove the protective cover over the syringe tip by twisting.
2. Insert the tip of the syringe into the hub of the needle. The needle may be held on by friction or by a locking mechanism. The fingers should be held well back from the point of attachment of the needle to the syringe.
3. Leave the needle guard in place until just before use. To remove the guard, pull it straight off or twist very gently.
4. To remove the needle from the syringe, insert the needle back into the needle guard and twist sharply.

When pulling back the plunger of the syringe, the fingers should not come in contact with any part of the plunger except the flat knob at the end. The barrel of the syringe should be held in the other hand, as shown in figure 9.1. Contamination of the medication can occur in some procedures if the plunger is touched with the fingers. This problem is more common when working with vials than with ampules because fluid is drawn into the syringe at least twice—once for the diluent and once for the reconstituted drug. It is a good practice to develop a technique that can be used safely in all situations.

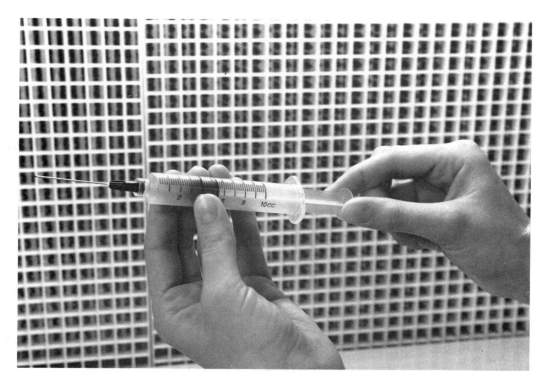

FIGURE 9.1. PULLING BACK THE SYRINGE PLUNGER

A common problem in withdrawing medication is that air may also be drawn into the syringe. The presence of air bubbles in a syringe prevents accurate measurement of the solution. To remove air bubbles from a syringe:

1. Hold the syringe in a vertical position so that the needle is pointing upward.
2. Pull the plunger back a short distance so that some air enters the syringe and solution is drawn in from the needle.
3. Firmly tap the barrel of the syringe with the fingers or knuckles so that air bubbles clinging to the side are freed and float to the top of the syringe.
4. Expel all the air in the syringe by slowly pushing in the plunger until the solution is at the tip of the syringe.
5. Read the volume of solution by aligning the rubber end of the plunger with the graduation marks on the barrel of the syringe (figure 9.2).

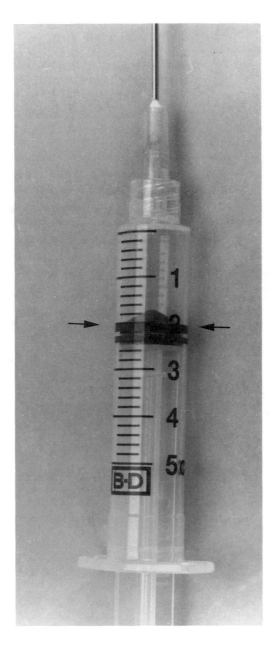

FIGURE 9.2. READING VOLUME OF SOLUTION IN SYRINGE

TRANSFERRING DRUGS FROM AMPULES USING A NEEDLE AND SYRINGE

An *ampule* (figure 9.3) is a small glass container sealed to preserve the sterility of an injectable solution. A colored stripe around the neck or more toward the top of an ampule indicates that the neck has been weakened to facilitate opening. An ampule should always be broken open at the neck, regardless of where the stripe is located.

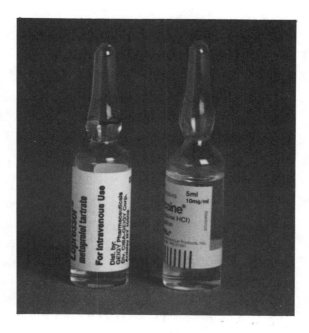

FIGURE 9.3. AMPULE

To open an ampule:

1. Hold the ampule upright and tap the top to remove solution in the head space.
2. Swab the neck of the ampule with an alcohol swab. This procedure does not make the outside of the ampule sterile, but it does serve as a disinfectant to reduce contamination.
3. Grasp the ampule on each side of the neck with the thumb and index finger of each hand.
4. Quickly snap the ampule as shown in figure 9.4. If the ampule does not snap easily, rotate it slightly so that pressure is exerted at a weaker point.
5. Inspect the opened ampule for any particles of glass that might have fallen inside.

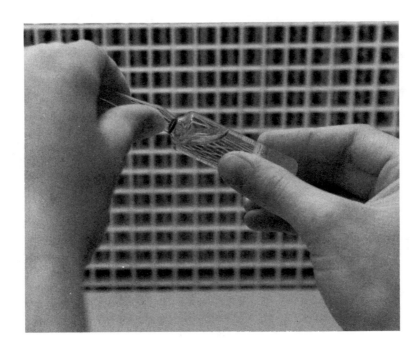

FIGURE 9.4. BREAKING OPEN AN AMPULE

To transfer the drug solution from an ampule:

1. Tilt the ampule to about a 20-degree angle.
2. Insert the needle into the ampule as shown in figure 9.5, taking care not to touch the ampule with the needle point around the neck where it is broken.

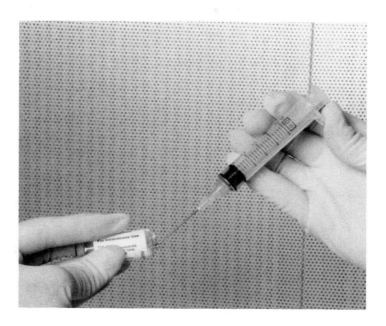

FIGURE 9.5. POSITION OF NEEDLE WITHIN THE AMPULE

3. Position the needle in the shoulder area of the ampule.
4. Pull the plunger back with the thumb and index finger (figure 9.6, method A) or push it up with the thumb of the same hand in which the syringe is held (figure 9.6, method B). Another method is to hold the ampule and barrel of the syringe in the same hand and pull the plunger back with the thumb and index finger of the other hand (figure 9.6, method C). Regardless of which method is used, it is important to maintain a clear pathway between the HEPA filter and the area where the aseptic procedure is performed. Hands, especially, should not obstruct this pathway.

METHOD A

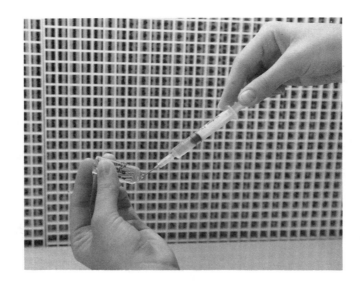

METHOD B

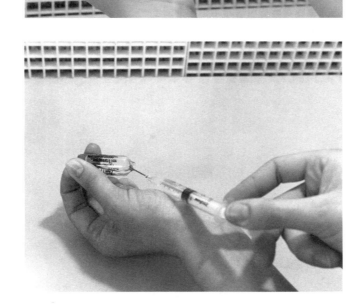

METHOD C

FIGURE 9.6.THREE METHODS OF REMOVING DRUG FROM AN AMPULE

USING FILTERS

It is common practice to filter drugs as they are drawn up from glass ampules in order to remove any glass fragments that may have fallen into the drug solution when the ampule was broken. A clarifying filter with a pore size of 5 microns is adequate for this purpose. The technique used to filter the solution depends on the type of filter used.

A stainless steel depth filter needle such as that shown in figure 8.19 is attached to the tip of the syringe. This filter, contained in the hub of the needle, is rigid enough so the solution may be filtered either as it is pulled into or expelled from the syringe—but not both ways in the same procedure. If the drug solution is to be filtered as the solution is pulled into the syringe, the following steps are used:

1. The filter needle is attached to the syringe.
2. The solution is pulled into the syringe.
3. The filter needle is removed.
4. A new needle is attached to the syringe.
5. The solution is expelled from the syringe.

Solutions may also be filtered using a membrane filter. These filters are used for a variety of purposes in various industries, so different filters are available for filtering different types of solutions. The appropriate filter should be selected to filter drug solutions. Because a membrane filter is supported only on the bottom, it can be used to filter a solution only as it is expelled from a syringe. The procedure is somewhat different from that described above for a stainless steel filter needle:

1. A regular needle is attached to the syringe.
2. The solution is pulled into the syringe.
3. Air bubbles are removed from the syringe as previously described.
4. The needle is removed from the syringe.
5. A membrane filter is then attached to the syringe.
6. A regular needle is placed on the end of the filter.
7. Air is eliminated from the filter chamber by holding the syringe in a vertical position so that the needle is pointing upward. Expel all the air in the filter chamber by slowly pushing in the plunger. Air must be expelled before the filter becomes wet; otherwise, the air will not pass through the filter. Do not pull back on the plunger when the membrane filter is being used. Because it is supported on only one side, the filter may rupture.
8. Once pressure is applied to expel air and solution from the system, pressure should be continuously applied.

Because using the membrane filter is more expensive and provides less flexibility than the stainless steel filter, the latter may be the recommended procedure for clarifying drug solutions withdrawn from ampules. However, a membrane filter with a pore size of 0.22 microns must be used to sterilize a solution by filtration.

TRANSFERRING DRUGS FROM VIALS USING A NEEDLE AND SYRINGE

Vials are glass containers sealed by a rubber closure covered with a protective aluminum band. An aluminum tab or plastic flip-off tab must be removed to insert the needle through the rubber closure. Some rubber closures are thin, soft, and pliable, whereas others are thick, hard, and brittle. *Coring*, or the breaking off of small pieces of the rubber closure when it is punctured by a needle, is much more prevalent with the latter.

The drug inside the vial may be in powder or liquid form. If the drug is in powder form, an extra step—*reconstitution*—must be performed before it can be added to the I.V. solution. Diluents such as sterile water for injection, bacteriostatic water for injection, or bacteriostatic 0.9% sodium chloride injection are usually used to reconstitute powdered drugs. The volume of a suitable diluent is specified in the package insert and frequently on the vial itself.

To reconstitute and transfer a drug from a vial:

1. Remove the protective tab and swab the top surface of the rubber closure of each vial with a disinfecting agent such as 70% isopropyl alcohol. Individually wrapped alcohol swabs are recommended.
2. Determine the correct volume of suitable diluent to reconstitute the powdered drug.
3. Using a needle and syringe, inject a volume of air equal to the volume of solution to be removed from the diluent vial, then remove the diluent from the vial.

Whenever a liquid is withdrawn from a vial, an equal volume of air should first be injected. For example, if 2 mL of solution is to be withdrawn from a vial, 2 mL of air should be injected first. This prevents a vacuum from being created in the vial. Alternatively, vented needles may be used, in which case the dynamics of air pressure can be disregarded.

Hold the diluent vial in an inverted position in one hand so that the other hand is free to pull back the plunger, as shown in figure 9.7. The needle should just penetrate the rubber closure to allow all of the solution to be withdrawn.

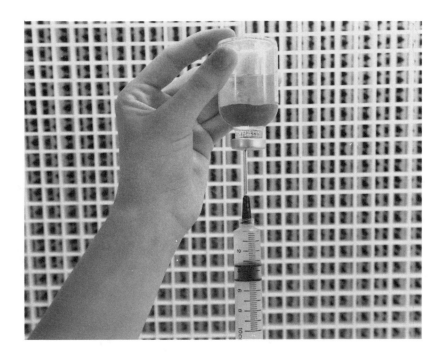

FIGURE 9.7. REMOVING SOLUTION FROM A VIAL

4. Inject the diluent into the medication vial.
5. Unless shaking is not recommended, remove the needle and shake the vial until the drug is dissolved. Immune globulin, for example, is not to be shaken because it causes foaming.
6. Reinsert the needle and remove the proper volume of drug solution. Do not inject air before withdrawing the drug solution at this point unless air was withdrawn before the needle was removed (step 5, above).
7. Remove all air bubbles from the syringe so the volume can be read accurately.

(*Note*: If the drug is already in liquid form, the term *drug vial* is substituted for the term *diluent vial* in step 3. Steps 2, 4, 5, and 6 are then unnecessary.)

To insert a needle through the rubber closure:

1. Lay the needle on the surface of the rubber closure so that the opening of the needle point is facing upward (figure 9.8).

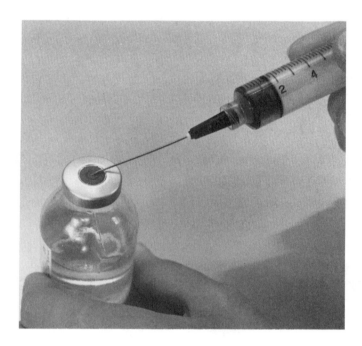

FIGURE 9.8. INITIAL POSITION OF NEEDLE TO ENTER A RUBBER CLOSURE

2. Exert downward pressure on the needle while rotating it upward. This action forces the rubber closure away from the bevel of the needle to minimize the chances of coring. The needle will penetrate the rubber at an angle (figure 9.9).

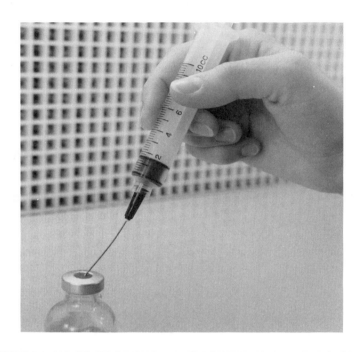

FIGURE 9.9. MOVEMENT OF NEEDLE WHILE PENETRATING RUBBER CLOSURE

DRUG TRANSFER TO A PLASTIC BAG

A syringe and needle are generally used to transfer a drug additive from a vial or ampule to a plastic bag. It is recommended that the needle gauge be not less than 19 to ensure resealing of the protective rubber cover. The needle must be at least ½ in. long to penetrate the inner diaphragm.

To transfer a drug additive to a plastic bag with a needle and syringe:

1. Remove the plastic I.V. from its outer wrap.
2. Assemble the needle and syringe.
3. Swab the mediation vial or ampule with a disinfecting solution and withdraw the necessary amount of drug solution. If the drug is in powder form, reconstitute it with the recommended diluent.
4. Swab the medication port of the plastic bag with a disinfecting solution.
5. Insert the needle into the medication port and through the inner diaphragm, as shown in figure 9.10. The medication port should be fully extended to minimize the chance of going through the side of the port.
6. Remove the needle.
7. Shake and inspect the admixture.

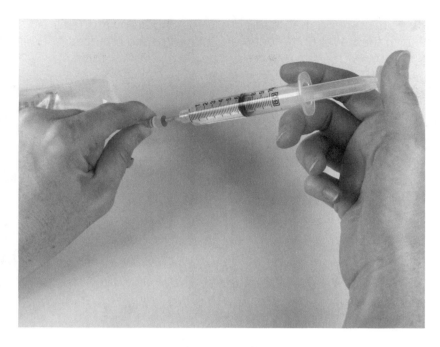

FIGURE 9.10. INJECTION OF DRUG INTO PLASTIC BAG WITH NEEDLE AND SYRINGE

INSPECTING COMPLETED ADMIXTURES

Each completed admixture must be inspected before it is delivered to the patient care area unit for administration. The following checks for accuracy must be made on every completed admixture to assure that the physician order, the label, and the components used are correct and in agreement:

1. The label is complete and free of errors.
2. The correct I.V. solution, including size and strength, has been used.
3. The correct drug additive(s), including strength and quantity, have been used.
4. The admixture is clear and free from particulate matter. This inspection is facilitated by holding the admixture in front of both light and dark backgrounds.
5. All drugs and solutions are within their labeled expiration dates.

BULK RECONSTITUTION

Reconstitution of powdered drugs is a time-consuming step in preparing I.V. admixtures when done on an individual basis. However, some high-use drugs are reconstituted or piggyback admixtures are prepared in bulk for greater efficiency. Enough doses of a drug to last an entire day may be prepared at one time. To make the process even more efficient, many pharmacists prepare enough doses in bulk to last several days and then freeze them, either as the reconstituted vial or as the completed admixture. Many drugs may be kept frozen until needed without altering their stability or potency. The frozen drugs are removed from the freezer several minutes before use to allow them to thaw at room temperature. Once thawed, the drugs should not be refrozen.

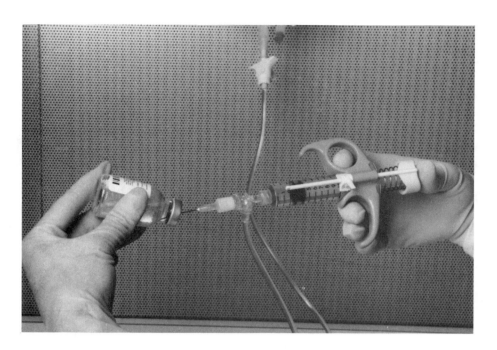

FIGURE 9.11. MASS RECONSTITUTION DEVICE

A mass reconstitution device (e.g., the Pharm-Aide Fluid Dispensing System) can be used for this purpose, as shown in figure 9.11. The device consists of a spring-loaded syringe attached to one end of a two-way valve. A length of tubing with a spike on one end is also attached to the two-way valve. The spike on the tubing is inserted into the solution container. As the plunger of the syringe is pulled back, solution from the container enters the syringe. As the plunger is pushed in, solution is forced out of the syringe and through the needle attached to the two-way valve. The plunger on the spring-loaded syringe can be adjusted to any volume of diluent and then locked at that position. Once the syringe is adjusted to deliver the desired volume to reconstitute the drug and the plunger is pushed in to expel the solution, the plunger automatically returns to the same place, allowing the same volume of diluent to enter the syringe repeatedly. The advantages of this system in terms of accuracy, control, and speed are substantial.

Mass reconstitution is performed with this device as follows:

1. Determine the volume of diluent to be added to each vial in order to produce the desired concentration.
2. Insert the spike of the mass reconstitution device into the proper site of the solution container serving as the diluent reservoir.
3. Hang the solution container from the rod across the top of the laminar flow hood.
4. Seal the valve on the syringe by turning the valve in a clockwise direction.
5. Attach a disposable needle to the two-way valve.
6. Pump the syringe until all air is removed from the tubing and syringe and the fluid path is primed with solution from the diluent reservoir.
7. Adjust the spring-loaded syringe to deliver the desired volume and lock into place. Check the plunger position and readjust if necessary. Monitor this position throughout the procedure.
8. Swab the rubber closures of the drug vials.
9. Inject the desired volume of diluent into the medication vial, using aseptic technique.
10. Release the thumb grip and allow sufficient time for the return spring to refill the syringe completely to the desired level.
11. Remove the needle from the medication vial and shake the vial until the drug is dissolved.

12. Repeat steps 9, 10, and 11 for subsequent vials, changing the needle on the two-way valve every 10 vials.
13. Inspect each vial for particulate matter and to assure that the medication is completely dissolved.

As an alternative to the mass reconstitution device just described, several dispensing pumps are available for mass reconstitution and bulk preparation (e.g., Baxa pump). Although these devices generally require calibration and programming prior to operation, significant efficiencies are gained through automating the bulk preparation process.

The mass reconstitution device or its equivalent has several uses in an admixture program, which include the following:

- Mass reconstitution of *powdered drugs for injection*, as shown in figure 9.11. Each vial of drug can be efficiently reconstituted with sterile water for injection or other recommended diluent, and either used immediately or frozen.

- Bulk preparation of *piggyback admixtures*. Bulk pharmacy containers that contain 20 or more doses of some commonly used antibiotics are available. The reconstituted drug in these bulk packages may be used as the solution reservoir and as a mass reconstitution device used to inject the drug into minibags very efficiently.

- Mass reconstitution of *piggyback containers supplied by the drug manufacturer*. These containers, usually made of glass and similar to minibottles without an air tube, contain one dose of a particular drug. Pharmacy personnel simply dilute the drug with the appropriate volume of the recommended diluent, label it, and send it to the patient care area for administration. Essentially, the pharmacy adds the solution to the drug, rather than performing the more common procedure of adding the drug to an I.V. solution.

PREMIXED ADMIXTURES

Many organizations are now purchasing premixed I.V. admixtures (figure 9.12) from manufacturers in order to save compounding time, eliminate the potential for contamination, reduce the potential for product waste, and reduce the potential for medication errors. Many high-use drugs are available premixed from manufacturers in standard doses and diluents. Premixed products are specially formulated and designed with longer stabilities than traditionally compounded products. These products are stored at room temperature or frozen, depending on drug stability. Examples of premixed admixtures stored at room temperature include a wide spectrum of potassium chloride solutions, antibiotics such as genta-micin, and large-volume admixtures such as dobutamine. Examples of frozen admixtures include many of the antibiotics in minibags.

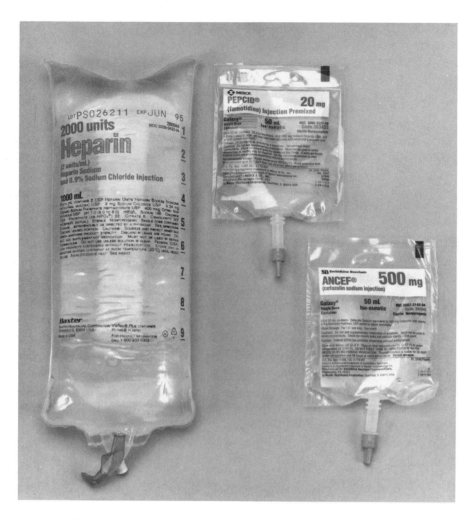

FIGURE 9.12. PREMIXED AND FROZEN PREMIXED I.V. ADMIXTURES

Dispensing premixed drugs involves simply thawing (if necessary), labeling, and checking. Frozen, premixed drugs should be passively thawed at refrigerator or room temperature. This may be facilitated using the air flow from a conventional fan or laminar flow hood. Microwave ovens and water baths are not recommended.

READY-TO-MIX, NURSE-ACTIVATED SYSTEMS

Ready-to-mix systems, such as the Abbott ADD-Vantage and the Baxter Mini-Bag Plus (figure 9.13), consist of a specially designed minibag with an adapter for attaching a drug vial. Connecting the drug vial to the minibag requires aseptic technique; therefore, these systems are typically assembled in a laminar flow hood within the pharmacy I.V. admixture area. Pharmacy dispenses these units with the unreconstituted drug vial attached to the minibag. The unit is fully labeled, but not mixed. Drug reconstitution takes place just prior to administration: To activate the system, the nurse breaks a seal or pulls a plug between the vial adapter and the minibag to reconstitute and transfer the drug from the vial to the minibag.

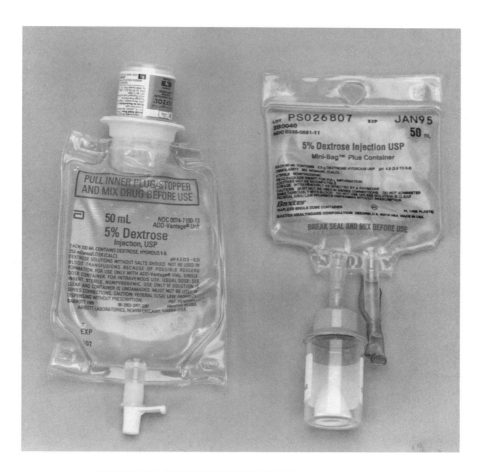

FIGURE 9.13. READY-TO-MIX NURSE-ACTIVATED SYSTEMS

The advantages of ready-to-mix systems include: (1) a significant reduction in product waste, because the drugs are not reconstituted until immediately prior to use; (2) reduced compounding time in pharmacy; and (3) decreased potential for medication errors, because the drug vial remains attached to the minibag. Disadvantages include: (1) increased product costs; (2) a potential failure to activate the system properly, so that the patient may receive only the diluent or a partial dose; and (3) the introduction of another "system" that personnel must learn.

CHAPTER 10

PARENTERAL NUTRITION SOLUTIONS

Parenteral nutrition solutions are complex admixtures used to provide nutritional support to patients who are unable to take in adequate nutrients via the gastrointestinal tract. These admixtures are composed of such energy sources as dextrose and fat, protein, electrolytes, vitamins, trace elements, and water. Parenteral nutrition solutions can be formulated so that they meet individual nutritional requirements based upon disease state, as well as metabolic and fluid status. Parenteral nutrition solutions are sometimes referred to as *total parenteral nutrition* (*TPN*) solutions or as *hyperalimentation* solutions. The latter is an older term that is not entirely accurate, but nonetheless is commonly used.

INDICATIONS FOR USE

Parenteral nutrition support is indicated for the nourishment of patients who are already malnourished or have the potential of becoming malnourished, and who are not able to take in adequate nourishment orally or from enteral nutritional support.

Examples of conditions under which parenteral nutrition may be used include the following diseases when the gastrointestinal tract may be partially or totally nonfunctional:

- Massive bowel surgery, such as short-bowel syndrome
- Conditions requiring bowel rest, such as acute *pancreatitis* (inflammation of the pancreas) or certain inflammatory bowel diseases
- Malnutrition, such as malnourished patients undergoing major surgery, or anorexia associated with cancer or cancer therapy (chronic vomiting or diarrhea)
- Hypermetabolic states, such as major trauma, critical illness, or burns in which the body uses more energy

Parenteral nutrition generally should not be initiated in patients who have a functional gastro-intestinal tract capable of absorbing nutrients. Also, it should not be initiated in patients who will need it for less than five days. Therapy may continue several days or weeks in hospitalized patients. Patients have been maintained on parenteral nutrition at home for several weeks to several years.

SOLUTION COMPOSITION

Parenteral nutrition solutions can be very complex, consisting of several components. The base solution consists of an amino acid solution (a source of protein), a dextrose solution (a source of carbohydrate calories), and sometimes an I.V. fat emulsion (a source of fat calories and essential fatty acids). These solutions, sometimes referred to as *macronutrients*, make up most of the volume of a parenteral nutrition solution.

Sterile water injection is commonly added to adjust the volume of the solution. For example, if 1 L of TPN solution is prescribed and the components make up only 900 mL, then 100 mL of sterile water is added to make up the final volume.

Intravenous fat (lipid) emulsion is required as a source of essential fatty acids. It is also used as a concentrated source of calories. Fat provides nine calories per gram, compared to 3.4 calories per gram provided by dextrose. I.V. fat emulsion may be admixed into the TPN solution with amino acids and dextrose, or piggybacked into the TPN line. When I.V. fat emulsion is admixed with the base solution, the resulting solution is referred to as a *total nutrient admixture* (*TNA*), or a *three-in-one admixture*. Admixing the fat emulsion with the base solution has become more common in recent years.

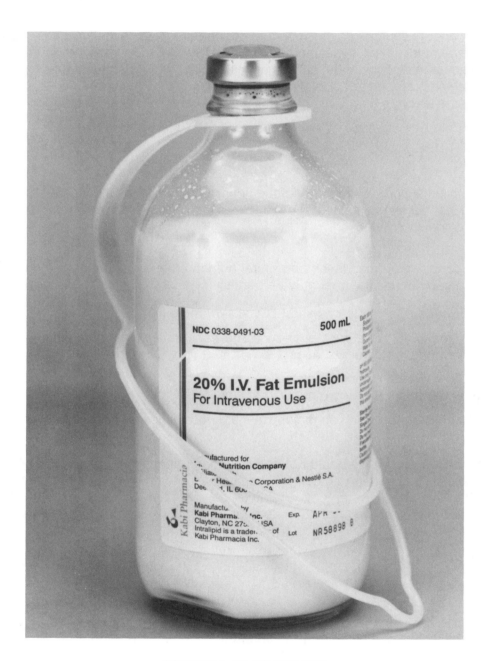

FIGURE 10.1. I.V. FAT EMULSION

Several electrolytes, trace elements, and multiple vitamins (collectively referred to as *micronutrients*) may be added to the base solution to meet individual patient requirements, usually determined by clinical laboratory data such as blood levels of electrolytes and clinical evaluation. Common electrolyte additives include sodium chloride (or acetate), potassium chloride (or acetate), calcium gluconate, magnesium sulfate, and sodium (or potassium) phosphate. Multiple vitamin preparations containing both water-soluble and fat-soluble vitamins are usually added on a daily basis. A trace element product containing zinc, copper, manganese, selenium, and chromium may be added as a standard trace element package. Other additives that are used less often and are more patient-specific include vitamin K, regular insulin, and histamine antagonists (e.g., cimetidine, ranitidine, famotidine).

Special formulations of amino acid solutions are available to meet the special requirements of patients with kidney (renal) or liver (hepatic) diseases. These products (e.g., RenAmin, Hepatamine) are formulated by varying the types and amounts of amino acids to meet the special requirements of these patients.

SOLUTION ADMINISTRATION

Because parenteral nutrition solutions are hypertonic, they must be administered with caution. Two primary means are used to administer parenteral nutrition solutions intravenously: through a central vein or through a peripheral vein.

Parenteral nutrition solutions are most commonly infused into a large central vein that leads directly to the heart (figure 10.2). The subclavian vein, the large vein under the collar bone (*clavicle*), is used most often. An incision is made through the skin and a central venous catheter is threaded through the subclavian vein until its tip is positioned just before the entrance to the heart. The solution exiting the tip of the catheter is diluted rapidly by the extensive blood flow.

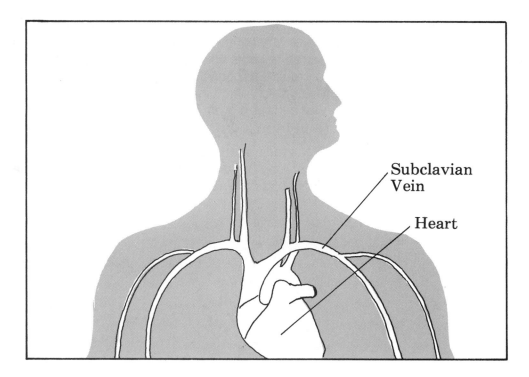

FIGURE 10.2. ADMINISTRATION OF A PARENTERAL NUTRITION SOLUTION THROUGH A CENTRAL VEIN

Parenteral nutrition solutions administered peripherally are usually used as a supplemental source of protein and calories for patients who are able to take some nutrition orally. Because they are approximately isotonic, I.V. fat emulsions can be administered either peripherally or centrally.

The concentration of parenteral nutrition solutions that can be infused safely through a peripheral vein (e.g., in the arm) is much less than that which can be administered through a central vein. For example, a 10% dextrose solution is generally regarded as the highest concentration of dextrose that should be administered through a peripheral vein, whereas concentrations of 25% or more may be given through a central vein. A peripheral vein is more easily damaged by a hypertonic solution than a central vein because, as a smaller vein, it has less blood flow.

To assure their accurate delivery, both central and peripheral nutrition solutions are almost always administered with an I.V. infusion pump. Parenteral nutrition solutions are commonly administered through an in-line filter in the administration set positioned as close to the patient as possible. However, I.V. fat emulsions—either alone or as part of a TNA solution—can be administered through an in-line filter only if it has a pore size of 1.2 micron or larger. An alternative is to piggyback the I.V. fat emulsion into the primary line below the in-line filter.

STARTING AND STOPPING THERAPY

Parenteral nutrition therapy should be initiated slowly, then the rate should be gradually increased to a therapeutic level or to the goal infusion rate. Gradually increasing the TPN rate prevents an increase in dextrose levels (*hyperglycemia*). For example, the solution may be initiated at 40 mL/hour and then increased by increments of 20 mL/hour to the goal infusion rate. This type of tapering gives the patient a chance to adjust to the increasing dextrose load. Serum glucose (dextrose) levels should be monitored frequently during the initiation of therapy. Assessment of each patient's response to the increase in rate is crucial.

Patients are usually started on oral feeding or enteral nutrition as their gastrointestinal function returns and their condition improves. Parenteral nutrition may be discontinued when the patient is receiving about 50 percent of his or her required calories via the oral, or enteral, route. Parenteral nutrition is usually discontinued gradually to prevent hypoglycemia (low blood glucose levels), which can be caused by abrupt discontinuation. The rate at which the TPN solution is discontinued depends upon the patient's status. Stable patients may be tapered off TPN solutions over as little as two hours.

The situation may exist in which the TPN solution must be stopped suddenly in patients who are not taking in adequate amounts orally or by enteral support. If this occurs, a 10% dextrose infusion should be started at the same rate as the TPN solution was running until the patient's status can be reevaluated.

Standardized Solutions and Order Forms Some hospitals and home care agencies have one or more standard base solution formulas that are used most commonly in the institution. Unless it would be highly inappropriate for a specific patient, the physician usually prescribes one of the standard base solutions and then tailors it to the individual patient needs with appropriate electrolytes. Some hospitals and home care agencies also use a special order form on which parenteral nutrition solutions must be prescribed. The advantages of standardizing solution formulas and order forms include the following:

1. Standardization ensures that all nutritional elements are provided to the patient, with less chance for omissions.
2. The intent of the prescribing physician is made clear, thus reducing the potential for medication errors and the number of calls a pharmacist must place to a physician to clarify orders.
3. The pharmacy can prepare base solutions in batches, thus improving efficiency and response time to new orders.

Nutrition Support Teams A nutrition support team is usually composed of a physician, a pharmacist, a dietitian, and a nurse. The responsibilities and authority of the parenteral nutrition team vary significantly from hospital to hospital. The team may represent a consultative service that sees patients only upon the request of an attending physician. In this situation, the team may actually write orders for the patient or may simply advise the attending physician on therapy. A second model is a team that follows all patients receiving parenteral nutrition and intervenes as needed to suggest changes in therapy to the attending physician. A third model is a team given the responsibility and authority to manage the therapy of all patients requiring nutrition support, including writing all orders for parenteral nutrition solutions.

The advantages of a nutrition support team include the following:

1. The quality of patient care is safeguarded through the expertise of each member of the team.
2. Greater coordination and efficiency in all aspects of patient care and order processing are promoted through better communication among the involved disciplines.
3. Consistent patient care is assured through centralized control and accountability.

The role of the clinical pharmacist on the nutrition support team is twofold. First, the pharmacist provides a vital communication link between the team prescribing the solution and the pharmacy staff compounding it. Second, the clinical pharmacist provides valuable input relating to drug incompatibilities, drug stability, and drug product selection.

24-Hour Solutions Rather than compounding two or three 1-L bags of parenteral nutrition solution daily for each patient, many health system pharmacies now provide parenteral nutrition solutions in a single 24-hour bag for each patient. This saves compounding time for the pharmacy and administration time for the nurse. Using 24-hour bags also improves the clarity of orders because only one order per day must be written, understood, and processed rather than two or three orders daily for each patient. Nutritional needs are usually thought of in terms of daily requirements, which is consistent with a daily order. One disadvantage is that if the solution is discontinued shortly after a 24-hour bag is hung, the potential waste can be significant.

Total Nutrient Admixtures (Three-in-One Solutions) As noted previously, parenteral nutrition base solutions usually consist of an amino acid solution and a dextrose solution. I.V. fat emulsions may be piggybacked into the parenteral nutrition solution line. Alternatively, combining all components into the same I.V. bag to create a total nutrient admixture (TNA, or three-in-one solution) simplifies admixture administration for nurses and decreases the hypertonicity of the solution being administered, making it better tolerated by the patient.

TNAs have several practical and clinical advantages over the traditional method of administering I.V. fat emulsion as a piggyback solution with the TPN solution. Combined with 24-hour bag systems and automated compounding, TNAs simplify the administration of TPN, resulting in time savings for nursing and pharmacy personnel. Clinically, the TNA allows for the infusion of I.V. fat emulsion over 24 hours, thus preventing the side effects associated with their rapid infusion over 6-8 hours.

PROBLEMS ASSOCIATED WITH ADMINISTERING PARENTERAL NUTRITION SOLUTIONS

Proper placement of the central venous catheter is vitally important for proper solution administration and should be confirmed by a chest X-ray before therapy is initiated. Common adverse effects associated with the administration of parenteral nutrition solutions include the development of infection in a small percentage of patients, which demands meticulous care of the catheter site. Another potential problem is *phlebitis* (inflammation of the vein), as the solutions can be very irritating because of their hypertonicity.

PROBLEMS ASSOCIATED WITH COMPOUNDING PARENTERAL NUTRITION SOLUTIONS

Compounding parenteral nutrition solutions can be very time consuming because of the need to prepare complex base solutions and numerous drug additives. Extensive calculations may be involved in determining the composition of the base solution as well as determining the amount of each drug to be added to the solution. Besides being time consuming, the potential for error must be recognized when the compounding process is so complex and so many calculations must be performed.

Some electrolytes prescribed in the parenteral nutrition solution may be incompatible when combined in high concentrations. These electrolytes, most notably magnesium or calcium combined with phosphate, should be maximally diluted and thoroughly mixed before being combined in these solutions to minimize the chance of precipitation.

The order of mixing is also important in total nutrient admixtures that combine the I.V. fat emulsion in the same bag with the amino acid and dextrose solutions. The dextrose and fat emulsion should not be directly combined. The order of mixing should be to add the amino acid to the fat, then add the dextrose.

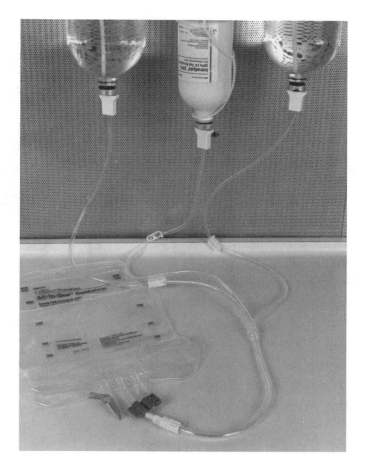

FIGURE 10.3. GRAVITY TPN TRANSFER SET

GRAVITY METHOD OF COMPOUNDING PARENTERAL NUTRITION SOLUTIONS

The gravity method of compounding these solutions uses a special empty plastic bag with a preattached, multiple-lead transfer set (figure 10.3). Transfer sets typically have either two or three leads, or branches. Each lead of the transfer set is connected to a different source solution, i.e., dextrose, amino acids, and/or lipid emulsion. The desired volume of each solution entering the empty plastic bag is controlled by a clamp on each lead of the set.

The amino acid, dextrose, and lipid source solutions are hung from the horizontal bar at the top of the laminar flow hood, and the empty plastic bag is laid on the work surface, as shown in figure 10.3. The volume of solution transferred is measured as it leaves each of the source containers. After the desired amount of solution is transferred to the empty plastic bag, all roll clamps are closed. The transfer set tubing is folded over near where it joins the bag and is clamped with a metal clamp to prevent solution from leaking out (figure 10.4). The Y transfer set is then cut on the side of the clamp away from the bag.

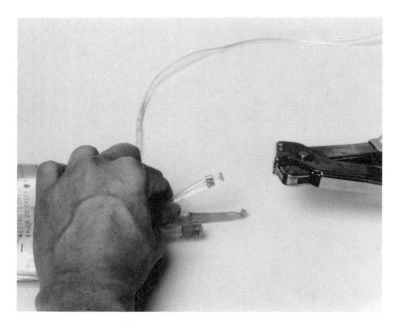

FIGURE 10.4. CLAMPING PREATTACHED TRANSFER SET

The gravity method of compounding is relatively inexpensive, in that high-technology equipment and supplies are not used. It does, however, have significant deficiencies when compared to other methods:

1. It is time consuming, in that solutions are not transferred by gravity quickly.
2. It is not very accurate, because solution volumes must be read from graduations on the sides of source solution containers.
3. It does not lend itself to easy pharmacist verification of solution volumes transferred.

However, when there are only a few parenteral nutrition solutions to compound on a daily basis, the gravity method is probably the most cost-effective and practical.

AUTOMIX COMPOUNDERS

If a pharmacy compounds a large number of parenteral nutrition solutions each day, the gravity method will prove much too time consuming. High-speed compounders are available to prepare complex nutrition support solutions safely, accurately, and quickly. The Automix 3+3 Compounder, which uses up to six source containers, is an example of such an automated device (figure 10.5).

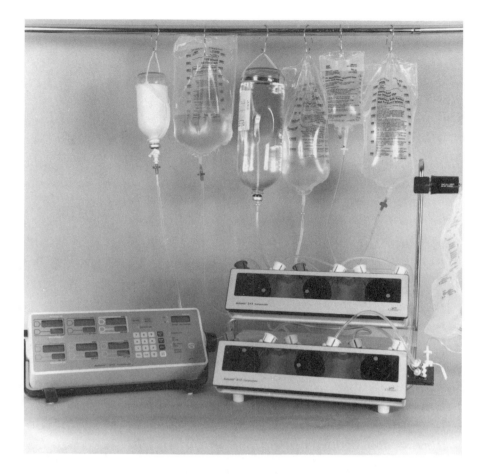

FIGURE 10.5. AUTOMIX 3+3 COMPOUNDER

A high-speed automated compounder offers at least three important advantages:

- Reduces the potential for touch contamination and provides the pharmacist with an accurate way to *verify* volumes transferred

- Provides *accuracy* within plus or minus 5% of the programmed volume for final volumes of 100 mL or more

- Provides *fast* transfer of solutions, mixing solutions at a rate of 1 L per 80 seconds

Pump Module The Automix Compounder consists of two principal parts—the pump module and the control module. The pump module, designed to be used inside a laminar flow hood, consists of hangers for six source containers, pump rotors that sequentially pump solution from the source containers to the final container, and a hanger for the final solution container (figure 10.6).

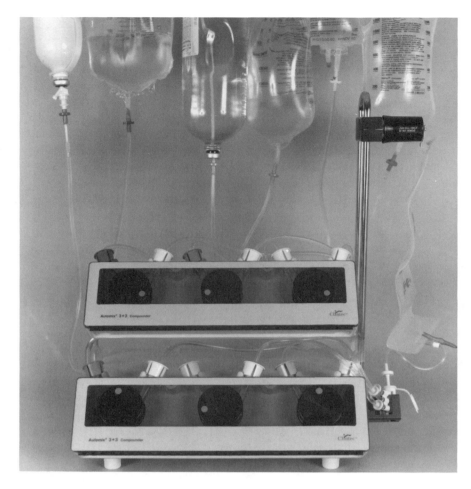

FIGURE 10.6. PUMP MODULE OF AUTOMIX 3+3 COMPOUNDER

All of these parts on the pump module are connected by a disposable six-station transfer set. Each lead of the transfer set connects a different source container to its respective station on the compounder. Each station is color-coded to match the color coding on the appropriate lead of the transfer set. At each station, the transfer set tubing is routed around the rollers of the pump rotor. All six leads of the transfer set come together at a common junction. Tubing from the final solution container is inserted into the transfer set junction. The final container hangs on a special hanger. The hanger connects to a precision electronic scale that measures fluid by weight. This is more accurate than measuring the fluid by volume because it is not adversely affected by air entering the system. Solution is transferred sequentially from each of the source containers into the final container.

Control Module The control module (figure 10.7) consists of the following parts:

- An operator panel with digital displays and a keypad to enter data regarding each station

- An internal microcomputer system for programming, controlling, and monitoring the compounding process

- Interface circuitry connecting the control module to the pump module and a host computer software program that controls the compounding process

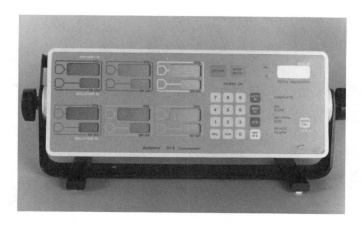

FIGURE 10.7. CONTROL MODULE OF AUTOMIX 3+3 COMPOUNDER

The control module is designed to be used outside the laminar flow hood. For each station corresponding to a different source solution, two pieces of data must be entered—the volume of that station's source solution to be transferred and the solution's specific gravity. *Specific gravity* is the relative weight of solution compared to water (1 g at 4°C). Thus, if 50% dextrose injection has a specific gravity of 1.17, it means that the weight of 1 mL is 1.17 times that of water. Specific gravity of each solution must be entered into the device because solution is transferred by weight, not by volume. The device does not measure volume directly, so the compounder monitors the weight of the final solution to determine the volume transferred. Thus, to transfer 1 mL of 50% dextrose injection, the compounder would transfer 1.17 g of that solution. If the specific gravity of each solution and the volume of the solution to be transferred into the final container are known, the required weight of the solution to be transferred can be determined by using the following equation:

$$\text{specific gravity (g/mL)} = \frac{\text{weight (g)}}{\text{volume (mL)}}$$

Compounding Audit System Some pharmacies have incorporated the use of a quality assurance feature into their automated compounding system to verify that the correct source solution container is attached to the correct lead of the transfer set. The lead of the transfer set and the source solution container both have small bar code labels attached. Bar code labels for transfer set leads are color-coded for efficiency and accuracy of setup. A hand-held laser bar code scanner/recorder (figure 10.8) is used to scan the bar code on the set and the solution. If the two bar codes match when scanned, the correct attachment is assured. Whenever the system detects a mismatch, it sounds an audible alarm, displays an on-screen warning message, and locks up until a supervisory level password is entered. All scanning operations are logged with user identification, time, and date. They can be reviewed on-screen or uploaded to a personal computer.

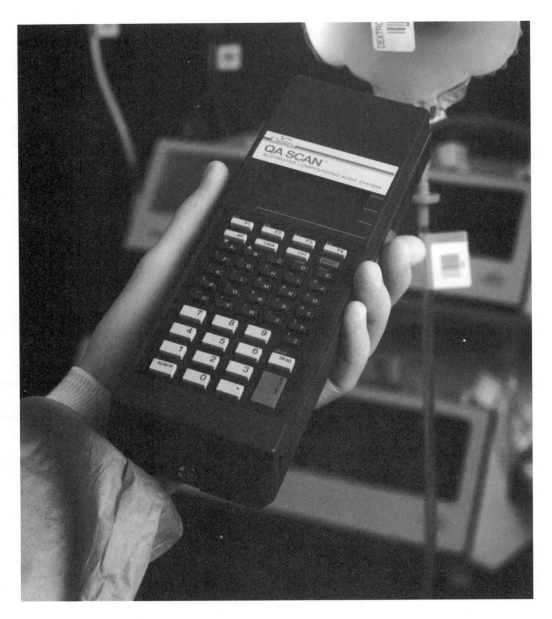

FIGURE 10.8. HAND-HELD SCANNER/RECORDER FOR AUTOMATED COMPOUNDING AUDIT SYSTEM

MULTITASK OPERATING SYSTEM SOFTWARE

The Multitask Operating System (MOS) is a microcomputer-based software program that allows the pharmacist additional control and flexibility when compounding parenteral nutrition solutions with the Automix and Micromix Compounders (figure 10.9).

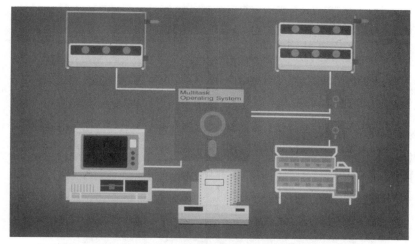

FIGURE 10.9. AUTOMIX AND MICROMIX COMPOUNDERS INTERFACED WITH PERSONAL COMPUTER AND MULTITASK OPERATING SYSTEM

The MOS program capabilities include the following:

1. Patient information and parenteral nutrition orders can be entered into the system. The data-base has a capacity for 300 patients and 1,500 individualized formulations.
2. The program performs calculations necessary for the compounding process.
3. Labels are generated individually or in batches, with a choice of label content and format. Bar-coding of labels is possible when using an appropriate printer.
4. Compounding instructions are transmitted to the compounder automatically.
5. Reports generated by the software include work load statistics, patient billing reports, inventory reports, and an activity log.

Advantages of the MOS software in the compounding process include accuracy, productivity, and a high level of flexibility. Potential for error is reduced because the software performs the necessary calculations, generates worksheets and labels, and automatically transfers prescription data directly to the compounder. These functions are done accurately through an automated system, and are done faster, thus improving productivity. Flexibility is also increased, because each MOS program can be customized by the user.

MICROMIX COMPOUNDER

Although the compounders and the software have greatly increased the efficiency with which parenteral nutrition base solutions can be compounded, they do not affect the time-consuming task of adding electrolytes, trace elements, and other drug additives. The Micromix Compounder is an example of a device that significantly reduces the time required to add these drugs to parenteral nutrition solutions (figure 10.10).

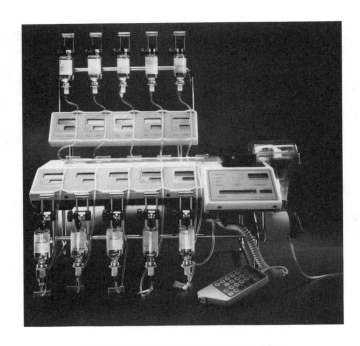

FIGURE 10.10. MICROMIX COMPOUNDER

The Micromix Compounder is designed to be operated inside the laminar flow hood and to be used in conjunction with the MOS software. It is capable of transferring to a final container selectable volumes between 0.3 mL and 650 mL from up to 10 source solution containers. The Micromix Compounder is similar to the Automix Compounder in that solutions are transferred by weight, not by volume.

Volume and specific gravity of the additives are automatically programmed by the MOS software. Whereas the Automix Compounders use pump rotors to move the solution through the transfer set, the Micromix Compounder induces a vacuum to draw solution from each source container into the final container.

The Micromix Compounder saves significant compounding time in the pharmacy. The device eliminates the need to prepare each drug additive in a syringe and have it checked by a pharmacist before adding it to the base solution. The MOS software calculates the volume of each additive to be delivered. The compounder enhances not only speed but safety. A single-piece 10-into-1 transfer set reduces the likelihood of operator touch contamination when multiple additives are handled. The automated transfer of multiple drug additives also eliminates any concern that syringes will get mixed up when doses are being prepared, and minimizes the potential for precipitate formation by automatically programming in a rinse between incompatible additives.

CHAPTER 11

CHEMOTHERAPY SOLUTIONS

METHODS OF CANCER TREATMENT

Cancer is a group of distinct diseases characterized by new, abnormal cellular growth (*neoplasm*), or tumor formation. In addition to tissue damage at the primary site, cancer may spread to distant parts of the body (*metastasize*). For example, colon cancer may metastasize to the liver.

The primary goal of therapy is to destroy the cancer cells or control their growth while minimizing the effect on normal cells. Relief of severe pain, nausea and vomiting, and other symptoms associated with the disease, in order to make the patient as comfortable as possible, is also an important goal of therapy.

Three primary methods are used in treating cancer: surgery, radiation therapy, and anticancer drugs. Each method has its place in therapy, depending on the type, location, and stage of the particular cancer. Each may be used alone or in combination with the others, again depending on the clinical situation.

Anticancer drugs are indicated in some localized cancers, as well as in such widespread cancers as leukemia and cancers that have metastasized to other organs. Some hormones and some drugs that modify the body's immune response are also categorized as anticancer drugs. However, most anticancer drugs are *cytotoxic* agents that preferentially kill fast-growing cells. Although the terms *cytotoxic drug*, *antineoplastic drug*, and *cancer chemotherapy drug* technically are used to describe different agents, the term *chemotherapy drug* will be used in this chapter to refer to all types of anticancer drugs.

CLINICAL USE OF CANCER CHEMOTHERAPY DRUGS

The clinical use and administration of cancer chemotherapy agents differ in several respects from usage patterns of most other drugs. To understand why seemingly unusual orders for chemotherapy drugs are received in the pharmacy, it may be helpful to review certain principles in the clinical use of these agents.

Chemotherapy drugs are frequently used together because combinations are generally more effective in killing cancer cells than are single agents. Also, chances that the cancer cells will become resistant to the drugs are lessened. By employing drugs that have different mechanisms of action and different toxicities, combination therapy can be used to obtain greater therapeutic effect with minimum toxicity. Thus, it is common to see orders for multiple chemotherapy drugs for the same patient.

Many cancer chemotherapy agents are administered on a cyclical, or intermittent, schedule. For example, certain combinations of drugs may be given weekly, monthly, or at other intervals. This allows more effective high-dose therapy to be given, followed by a minimally toxic, drug-free recovery period between treatments. This type of intermittent scheduling may continue for several months as long as the benefits outweigh the risks of treatment. Thus, it is common to see orders written for patients to receive chemotherapy agents intermittently, with several days or weeks elapsing between treatments. Many factors influence how chemotherapy agents are used in the clinical setting. Although high-dose intermittent therapy is common, low-dose continuous infusion may be indicated for certain drugs and clinical situations.

Another difference seen with chemotherapy agents is that they are more often administered I.V. push than are most other drugs. Thus, doses are commonly prepared in syringes as well as in large-volume infusions. Other routes of administration for chemotherapy agents may be encountered in an attempt to provide higher drug concentrations at the tumor site while minimizing toxicity. For example, drugs used to treat cancer of the central nervous system may be injected *intrathecally* (directly into the spinal cord fluid). Intrathecal injections must be prepared using preservative-free diluents to avoid serious adverse effects to the patient.

Most hospitals have a credentialing process that nurses must complete before they are permitted to administer drugs intravenously, and many hospitals require additional credentialing for nurses before they may administer chemotherapy drugs. During this process, nurses receive instruction and demonstrate their competence in the special precautions and administration techniques associated with chemotherapy drugs.

ADVERSE EFFECTS OF CHEMOTHERAPY SOLUTIONS

Important advances in the treatment of cancer have been made in recent years. However, patients often experience severe adverse reactions and side effects to chemotherapy when administered in therapeutic doses. Thus, toxicity is a major limiting factor in the use of chemotherapy agents and is the reason their use should be directed by an oncologist or other physician experienced in the treatment of cancer.

Adverse effects can be divided into those related to administration of the drug and those representing predictable side effects. Proper administration of chemotherapy drugs is essential because tissue damage can result if extravasation of the drug occurs. Some drugs, such as doxorubicin, must be administered with extreme caution. Regardless of the chemotherapy agent, treatment of extravasations should be initiated immediately in accordance with the established hospital policy.

Of the adverse side effects that are predictable with a specific drug, dose, or dosing schedule, the most common is nausea and vomiting. Most chemotherapy drugs cause this side effect, which may be severe and persistent. Other common side effects include loss of hair, sores inside the mouth and throughout the gastrointestinal tract, and changes in blood cell counts (red blood cells, which carry oxygen to tissues; white blood cells, which fight infections; and platelets, which stop bleeding).

PROBLEMS ENCOUNTERED IN SOLUTION PREPARATION

Preparing, storing, and disposing of chemotherapy agents has the potential to expose pharmacy personnel to substantial amounts of these drugs if they are not handled properly. The immediate effects of surface contact with a chemotherapy agent may be local tissue damage and extreme irritation to the skin, eyes, mouth, or nose. Of even greater concern is the long-term risk associated with handling these drugs. Although more research is needed, enough evidence exists to suggest that harmful effects could develop if unprotected workers are exposed to chemotherapy drugs over a long period, even at low doses.

The potential for exposure to chemotherapy drugs is greatest after spills or during manipulations that generate aerosol droplets of the solution. The latter occurs most commonly when personnel withdraw needles from vials, break ampules, expel air from drug-filled syringes, and transfer drugs with needles and syringes. The risk of exposure to an individual depends on two factors: the inherent toxicity of the particular drug (some drugs are more toxic than others) and the extent of the exposure. The risk includes consideration of the magnitude of a single exposure as well as cumulative exposure at low levels over a long period. Until additional facts are known, precautions must be taken during the preparation of these admixtures to protect the individual worker and the work environment, all the while maintaining the sterility of the product.

ENVIRONMENTAL PRECAUTIONS

The horizontal or vertical laminar flow hood commonly used in the preparation of I.V. admixtures should not be used in preparing chemotherapy drugs. Although they protect the drug product from microbial contamination, they do not protect personnel or the environment from the hazards of these agents. These laminar flow hoods blow air across the work surface toward the operator and into the work environment. Suspended drug particles or aerosols of chemotherapy agents thus can easily contaminate both workers and the work environment.

Although it may be obvious, it should be stated that a conventional laminar flow hood cannot simply be turned off and used as a clean place to compound chemotherapy drugs. First, the drug product is not protected from microbial contamination, since the hood is turned off. Second, and more important, if the laminar flow hood is contaminated—for example, if a drug is accidentally expelled from a syringe onto the HEPA filter—and then turned back on, the operator and the work environment will be continuously contaminated by the chemotherapy drug being blown outward by the laminar air flow.

Rather than using a horizontal laminar flow hood, it is recommended that a biological safety cabinet be used to provide protection for the worker, the work environment, and the drug (figure 11.1). A biological safety cabinet functions by having air taken into the unit at the top, where it passes through a prefilter to remove gross contaminants. Air then passes through a HEPA filter and is directed down toward the work surface just as with a vertical laminar flow hood. The filter forms the ceiling of the work area in the biological safety cabinet and removes bacteria to provide ultraclean air. Unlike in a vertical laminar flow hood, however, as air approaches the work surface, it is pulled through vents at the front, back, and sides of the unit (figure 11.2). A major portion of the contaminated air is recirculated back into the cabinet and a minor portion is passed through a HEPA filter before being exhausted into the room.

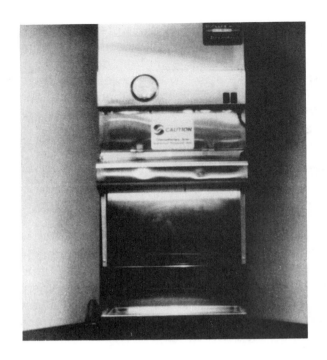

FIGURE 11.1. BIOLOGICAL SAFETY CABINET

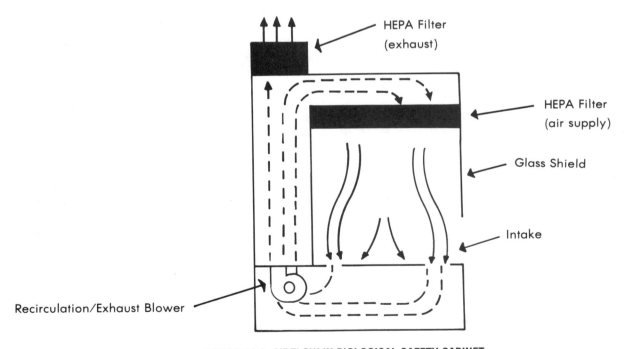

FIGURE 11.2. AIRFLOW IN BIOLOGICAL SAFETY CABINET

Biological safety cabinets are of two basic types. Class 2, type A (just described) represents the minimum recommended environment for preparing chemotherapy agents. Class 2, type B biological safety cabinets have greater intake flow velocities and are vented outside the building rather than back into the room. This type of safety cabinet is preferred, but the need to vent the filtered air to the outside can carry with it a substantial construction cost.

It is important that biological safety cabinets run continuously. If turned off for any reason (e.g., maintenance or changing the HEPA filter), the biological safety cabinet must be thoroughly cleaned with a detergent, and the exhaust area must be covered with impermeable plastic and sealed to prevent any contaminants from escaping from the unit.

DRESS PRECAUTIONS

In addition to working in a protected environment provided by a biological safety cabinet, it is essential that the individual take appropriate precautions to minimize inhalation or direct contact with chemotherapy drugs (figure 11.3).

Gowns Gowns should be worn to protect arms and clothes when chemotherapy solutions are prepared. Gowns should have a closed front and long sleeves with tight-fitting, elastic cuffs. The material should be made of a low-permeability, lint-free material. Washable gowns are not recommended because they are permeable to solutions and they may be a source of contamination when laundered. Once a gown is worn for a compounding procedure, it should not be worn outside the preparation area.

Gloves Disposable surgical latex gloves should always be worn when chemotherapy drugs are handled and should be changed at the beginning of preparing each batch of solutions. Although no glove material is impervious to all drugs, latex surgical gloves are recommended unless a drug manufacturer recommends another type of glove for a specific drug. These gloves easily permit double-gloving, which is recommended because it adds greater thickness without affecting manipulations. Glove thickness and time of exposure are the most important factors in limiting drug exposure. Care should be exercised to maintain a tight fit between the gloves and the gown cuffs.

Companies such as BioSafety Systems, Inc. (San Diego, California), have developed specialty products for use in chemotherapy procedures. High-quality latex gloves are available that feature added thickness and an extended cuff to provide maximum protection.

Eye Shields Eye shields are recommended if work is being done outside a biological safety cabinet or inside one that does not have a protective glass shield between the work area and the operator. Eyewash fountains or other eyewash alternatives should be immediately available in case chemotherapy solution is accidently splashed in the eye.

Masks Surgical masks do not provide protection against breathing aerosols. However, the operator may feel more secure wearing a surgical mask and eye shields for added protection and should be permitted that choice. Specialty dust/mist respirators are available for protection specifically when compounding chemotherapy solutions.

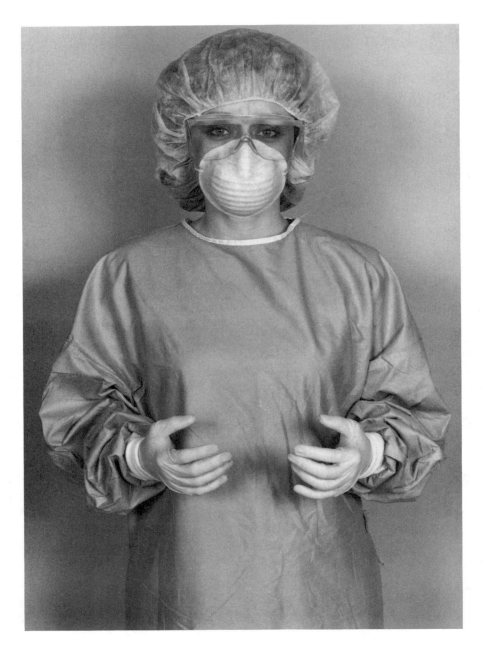

FIGURE 11.3. DRESS PRECAUTIONS FOR HANDLING CHEMOTHERAPY DRUGS

COMPOUNDING TECHNIQUE PRECAUTIONS

__Working in a Biological Safety Cabinet__ Proper aseptic technique is essential to protect the operator, the work environment, and the product. Principles of aseptic technique are the same as those for working in a vertical laminar flow hood. Preparation procedures should be well organized to avoid having to go in and out of the biological safety cabinet frequently. Commonly used supplies and materials needed for product preparation and for proper disposal should be readily available.

__Selecting Syringes__ Because Luer-Lok fittings are less likely to come loose, they are recommended over syringes in which the needle is held on by friction. The size of the syringe selected should be large enough so that when the drug is drawn into the syringe it will not be more than three-quarters full.

Manipulating Drugs in Vials Diluent should be added to the vial slowly. Alternately injecting small amounts of diluent and allowing an equal volume of displaced air to enter the syringe guards against problems resulting from excessive pressure in the vial. Once the diluent is added, a little more air should be withdrawn to create a slight negative pressure in the vial, thus decreasing the likelihood that aerosol droplets will be sprayed when the needle is withdrawn.

When a drug is withdrawn from a vial, air equal to the volume of solution to be withdrawn should be injected. Again, alternately injecting small amounts of air and allowing an equal volume of liquid to enter the syringe maintains the proper pressure inside the vial. Before the needle is withdrawn from the vial, drug from the needle and tip of the syringe should be cleared by drawing additional air into the syringe. As shown in figure 11.4, a sterile gauze pad should be wrapped around the needle and vial before the needle is withdrawn in order to avoid spraying aerosol droplets.

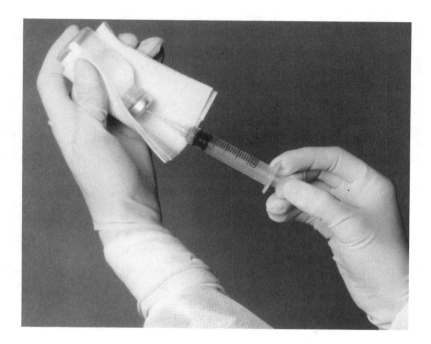

FIGURE 11.4. WITHDRAWING NEEDLE FROM VIAL

Manipulating Drugs in Ampules Any drug in the headspace of the ampule should be tapped down. A sterile gauze pad should be wrapped around the neck of the ampule before breaking in order to trap any aerosolized material or glass fragments.

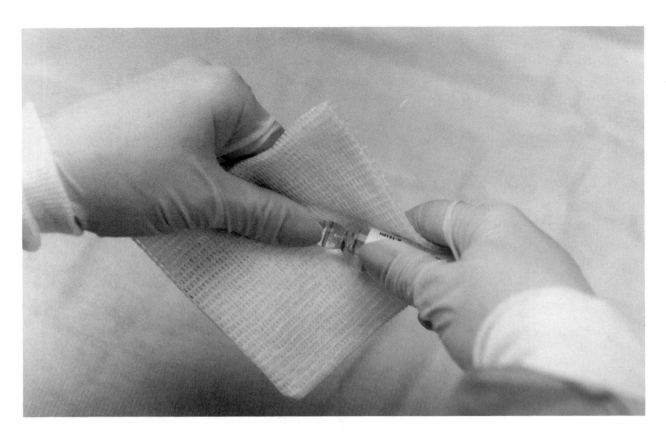

FIGURE 11.5. BREAKING AN AMPULE

Disposing of Excess Solution After drawing the drug into a syringe, it should be cleared from the needle and tip of the syringe by drawing additional air into the syringe. After any air bubbles are removed, excess solution should be returned to its original vial, an empty vial, or other suitable, closed container. Excess solution should not be expelled into an open container or into the air.

Selecting Needles Chemotherapy dispensing pins (figure 11.6) are venting devices that have a unique airflow design to allow solution to be safely withdrawn from a vial without aerosolization. Rather than building up pressure in the vial, air is allowed to escape the closed system through a 0.2 micron hydrophobic air-venting filter. The spike of the chemotherapy dispensing pin is inserted into the vial, and the syringe is inserted into the Luer-Lok attachment on the unit to allow solution to be withdrawn from the vial.

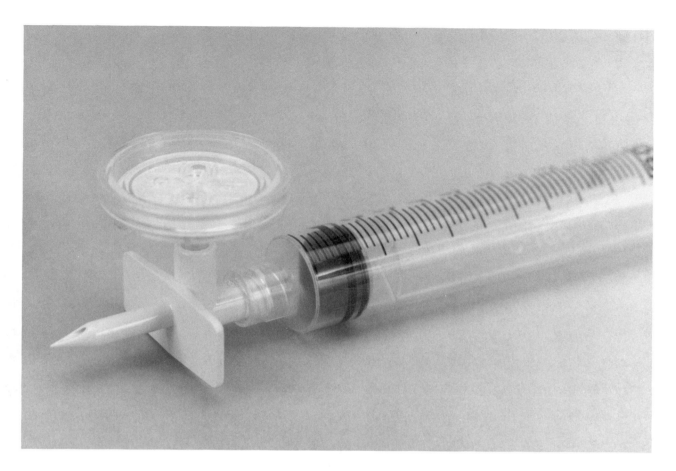

FIGURE 11.6. CHEMOTHERAPY DISPENSING PIN

___**Protecting the Work Surface**___ The work surface of the biological safety cabinet should be covered by a disposable, absorbent, plastic-backed liner (figure 11.7) to absorb any spilled solution. The liner should be changed at the end of each shift or when there is a noticeable spill. The liner has three layers: the top is a penetrable mesh; the second is an absorbent gauze, and the bottom is a nonpermeable plastic. If a spill occurs on the liner, it passes through the top layer and is absorbed into the second layer to maintain a dry work surface.

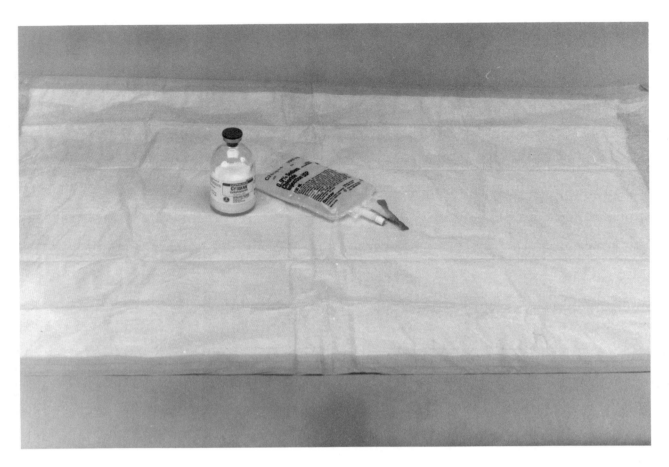

FIGURE 11.7. PROTECTIVE ABSORBENT PAD

__Assuring Proper Labeling__ Syringes or I.V. admixtures containing chemotherapy agents should have a distinctive supplemental label that reads "Caution: Chemotherapy—handle with gloves; dispose of properly."

__Packaging the Final Product__ The final chemotherapy product should be placed in a sealed container (e.g., zipper-locked plastic bag) for delivery to the patient care area in order to contain any spillage if the chemotherapy solution leaks from its container.

__Packaging Contaminated Materials__ Contaminated materials used in preparing chemotherapy solutions should be placed in sealable, leakproof, punctureproof containers before leaving the biological safety cabinet. Such materials may include needles, syringes, empty vials or ampules, and gauze pads. Needles should not be clipped or recapped in order to prevent aerosolization or accidental needle sticks.

A specialty recapping device is available that is simply a "well" to hold the removed needle guard in an upright position, similar to the way in which a desk pen is held in a penholder. When the needle is uncapped, the needle guard can be placed in the holder. After the syringe has been used, the needle, still attached to the syringe, can be reinserted into the needle guard held in place by the recapping device. Thus, syringes can be recapped without the danger of needle sticks.

__Washing Hands__ Operators should wash their hands not only before the compounding process but also after preparation of chemotherapy drugs.

DISPOSAL PRECAUTIONS

Discarded gloves, gowns, needles, and syringes used in preparing chemotherapy drugs present a possible source of contamination to housekeeping personnel and should be disposed of properly. These materials are considered to be hazardous waste and should be treated accordingly, following the institution's safety management policies. Receptacles should be conveniently located and properly labeled "Caution: Hazardous Chemical Waste." For easy identification, containers should be lined with a plastic bag of a color different from those of other trash bags used in the institution. Containers should be leakproof and punctureproof, and should be used exclusively for chemotherapy waste. Drug waste should be separated from other chemotherapy waste.

Nursing personnel face additional concerns over disposal of such materials as I.V. sets used in administering chemotherapy drugs. They must also be concerned with contaminated linen, blood, etc., from patients.

SPILLS AND BREAKAGE PRECAUTIONS

All staff members who handle chemotherapy drugs must be familiar with the institution's procedure for dealing with spills and personal exposure. This procedure should be posted in a conspicuous place. Spill kits that contain the necessary equipment and supplies to clean up spills should be purchased or assembled and made readily available wherever chemotherapy solutions are prepared or administered.

Spills should be cleaned up immediately by trained, protected personnel. For small spills, the person cleaning up should wear a gown, eye shields, and double gloves (an outer pair of utility gloves and an inner pair of latex gloves). Larger spills should be covered with an absorbent liner or a spill pillow, and the area should be restricted. Spills should be handled in a manner that does not generate aerosols. A respirator should be worn if aerosol droplets or airborne powder are likely to be generated during the cleanup.

If workers are personally contaminated, gowns and/or gloves should be changed immediately. Spills on the skin should be washed with soap. Contact with eyes should be followed by a five-minute eye wash. Medical attention should be sought immediately.

CHAPTER 12

FLOW OF ADMIXTURE ORDERS

Regardless of the specific procedures involved in a particular admixture system, certain steps must take place to assure accuracy in ordering, preparing, checking, delivering, and administering the admixture. The sequential steps involved in the order flow depends on the degree of computerization and the specific policies and procedures of the organization. This chapter outlines a typical sequence, although there could be many variations.

Flow Diagram for Admixture Orders

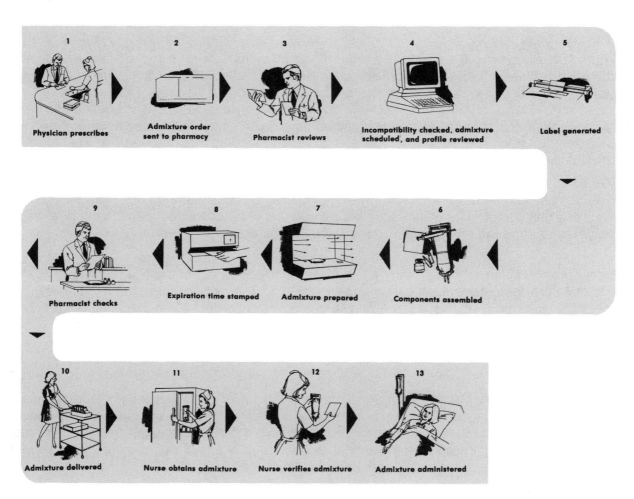

FIGURE 12.1.FLOW DIAGRAM FOR ADMIXTURE ORDERS (ADAPTED FROM GODWIN HN, SHOUP LK (BALCHIS GL, ED). *IMPLEMENTATION GUIDE: CENTRALIZED INTRAVENOUS ADMIXTURE PROGRAM.* DEERFIELD, IL: BAXTER HEALTHCARE CORP., 1977)

STEP 1—PHYSICIAN PRESCRIBES THE ADMIXTURE

A physician initiates the order for an admixture by writing the prescription on the physician order form as described in chapter 6. The prescription includes the patient's name and location; the drug name and dose; usually the solution, strength, and volume; the route, frequency, and rate of administration; the physician's signature; and the date and time the order was written.

Pharmacists may have considerable input into the I.V. admixture prescribed in some organizations. If the pharmacist actually writes the order, it is usually as a verbal order that the physician will countersign within 24 hours. As the use of computers in health care organizations increases, it is becoming more commonplace for physicians to enter the order directly into a computer system to update the electronic medical record.

STEP 2—NURSE REVIEWS ORDER AND SENDS TO PHARMACY

A nurse usually checks the physician's order for an I.V. admixture for completeness and determines when the doses will be scheduled for administration. Standard administration times are used in some organizations (e.g., q6h may mean that doses will be administered at 12 a.m.–6 a.m.–12 p.m.–6 p.m. or at 3 a.m.–9 a.m.–3 p.m.–9 p.m.), but they more commonly apply only to piggyback doses and not to primary solutions. In the absence of standardized administration times, the nurse should indicate the scheduled administration times and when the first dose is needed so that pharmacy personnel will know when the doses should be prepared.

In an effort to get the order to the pharmacy as quickly as possible, the nurse may not review the order first. The unit secretary or clerk sends the physician's order or a direct copy to the pharmacy by the quickest route, and the nurse uses the chart copy of the order for reference.

Orders may be sent to the pharmacy via courier, pneumatic tube, or facsimile machine. Orders may be entered into the computer system by the unit secretary or clerk, but a pharmacist must review the accuracy of the order entry against a direct copy of the physician order before preparing the admixture.

STEP 3—PHARMACIST REVIEWS THE ORDER

Upon receipt of the physician's order, a pharmacist checks it for completeness and appropriateness. Completeness means having all the necessary elements of the prescription order included and understandable. Appropriateness means checking for drug selection, dosage, compatibility, and administration directions. Questions about the completeness or appropriateness of an admixture order should be directed to the prescribing physician or the nurse, depending on the specific problem.

As the role of pharmacy technicians expands and they become more highly trained individuals, the pharmacist may be asked to review only unusual orders before the admixtures are compounded. Technicians can usually judge the completeness and appropriateness of routine orders, recognizing that orders for pediatric patients and oncology patients require more skill. A pharmacist is still required to check the completed admixture.

STEP 4—PHARMACIST OR TECHNICIAN ENTERS ORDER INTO SYSTEM

As mentioned in chapter 8, most admixture systems rely on the physician order's being entered into a computer system; the trend toward managed care will make it imperative that the pharmacy system be interfaced with the larger health care enterprise's computer system.

The physician's order may be entered by a pharmacist or by a technician with a pharmacist's verification. It is critical that a pharmacist verify the accuracy of the order entry, because subsequent doses of the admixture will be prepared based on information in the computer system. When the order is entered into the computer, the system can usually check for potential incompatibilities, schedule administration times, and review the patient's current medication profile for drug interactions. Order entry into a computer system will enable generation of labels for future doses, generation of patient charges for products administered, and accumulation of statistics and work load data for the department. Computerizing the order entry function provides a good screening system, but it does not eliminate professional judgments that the pharmacist must make in deciding whether an admixture will be safe and appropriate for a particular patient.

As previously mentioned, in some organizations medication orders may be entered into the computer system by a nurse or a unit secretary or clerk. In these situations, it is still imperative that a pharmacist review the physician's order or a direct copy to verify the accuracy of data entered.

Noncomputerized admixture systems exist only in very small programs. These operations typically use an admixture schedule card or similar document to build a profile on the patient and to know when a particular admixture is scheduled for administration. This card typically contains the patient's name and room number; the I.V. solution name and volume; the drug additive(s) name and quantity; administration schedule; rate of administration; date the order was written; the physician's name, if desired; and any special comments that relate to the particular admixture. An example of an admixture schedule card is shown as figure 12.2. The time at which the first admixture is scheduled for administration is written opposite the line for solution no. 1. After preparing the admixture, the technician initials the proper space following the corresponding solution number. The pharmacist providing the final check for accuracy of the admixture initials in the same space.

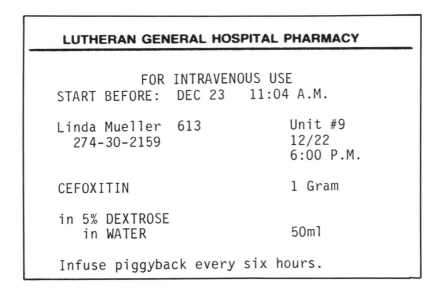

FIGURE 12.2. ADMIXTURE SCHEDULE CARD

STEP 5—TECHNICIAN GENERATES LABEL

Labels are prepared according to an established format described in the pharmacy's policy and procedure manual. An example is shown in figure 12.3.

LUTHERAN GENERAL HOSPITAL PHARMACY

```
                FOR INTRAVENOUS USE
START BEFORE:  DEC 23   11:04 A.M.

Linda Mueller   613          Unit #9
  274-30-2159                 12/22
                              6:00 P.M.


CEFOXITIN                    1 Gram

in 5% DEXTROSE
   in WATER                  50ml

Infuse piggyback every six hours.
```

FIGURE 12.3. ADMIXTURE LABEL

Typical I.V. admixture labels include the following information:

- Patient's first and last name
- Patient room number or location
- Drug additive name and dose
- Solution name, strength, and volume
- Date and time of scheduled administration
- Administration directions
- Expiration date and time, usually stated on the label as not more than 24 hours beyond the time of administration
- Preparation date (this is sometimes identified by the expiration date if a 24-hour stability dating is routinely used)
- Initials of person who prepared and/or checked the admixture

It is helpful to a nurse for the pharmacy to convert the administration rate to drops per minute for large-volume parenterals or for piggybacks that require a prescribed time for infusion. The conversion of milliliters per hour to drops per minute can be done automatically through the pharmacy computer system or is facilitated by the use of a conversion table. Conversion tables must be developed for a specific manufacturer of the administration set being used, because the number of drops per milliliter differs according to manufacturer.

Perhaps the greatest time saving realized in a computerized admixture system is in preparing labels. A technician or pharmacist need only request labels for a certain time interval and the computer will print all the admixture labels required during that period. The computer labels then become the working document that the technician consults in compounding the needed admixtures.

STEP 6—TECHNICIAN ASSEMBLES COMPONENTS

Admixtures with at least 24-hour stability are usually prepared in batches at regular intervals (e.g., three times a day), depending on the frequency of scheduled deliveries to the patient care areas. At the appropriate times, I.V. solutions, diluents, drug additives, syringes and needles, and labels (and schedule card if a noncomputerized system) are assembled on a plastic tray prior to preparation (figure 12.4).

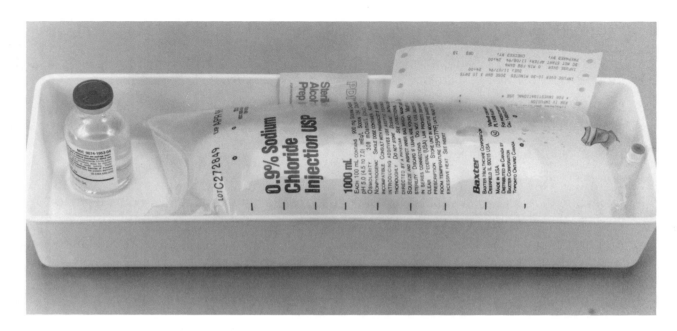

FIGURE 12.4. ADMIXTURE SETUP TRAY

The advantages of setting up each order on an individual tray are:

1. One order at a time can be taken into the laminar flow hood for compounding, thus keeping orders for different patients separated.
2. All of the components necessary for compounding the admixture are at hand so that a technician does not go into and out of the hood unnecessarily.
3. All of the components, including used medication vials, and the completed admixture can be reassembled onto the tray and placed on a counter outside the hood for the pharmacist to check.

STEP 7—TECHNICIAN PREPARES ADMIXTURE

One tray at a time is taken inside the laminar flow hood where the technician prepares the admixture. All I.V. admixtures must be prepared inside the hood using aseptic technique, as described in chapter 9. The admixture should be labeled as soon as the drug is added to the I.V. solution. Components used in preparing the admixture (i.e., syringe, used medication vials, etc.) should be placed back on the tray so that a pharmacist can check the final product. A sterile, tamperproof cap or seal may be placed on the solution container to assure the nurse that the admixture has not been tampered with since it was prepared.

STEP 8—EXPIRATION TIME STAMPED

The proper expiration date is stamped on the label with an automatic time clock (figure 12.5). The label is affixed to a plastic bag in the upright position below the printed identification in such a manner that the graduation marks on the side of the container remain visible (figure 12.6). The label is affixed to a solution bottle in an inverted position over the solution label so that it can be easily read when the bottle is hanging. Routinely, a 24-hour expiration date is stamped on admixture labels. However, if drugs are stable for shorter periods, the appropriate expiration time may be stamped on the label with a rubber stamp. Routinely using a 24-hour expiration date stamped on the label by an automatic time clock also provides documentation that the admixture was actually compounded 24 hours prior to the stamped date and time.

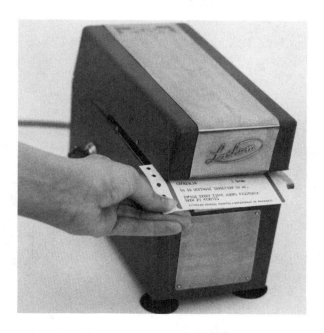

FIGURE 12.5. AUTOMATIC TIME CLOCK FOR STAMPING EXPIRATION DATE

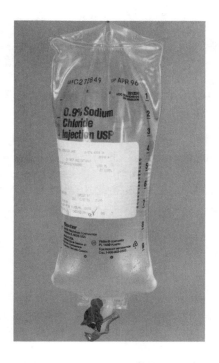

FIGURE 12.6. LABEL AFFIXED TO ADMIXTURE

A final check should be performed by the technician to see that the correct solution and additives have been used, that the label is complete and accurate, and that the admixture is clear and free of particulate matter. The technician then initials the label to document who prepared the admixture.

STEP 9—PHARMACIST CHECKS COMPLETED ADMIXTURE

The labeled admixture; used medication vials or ampules; and needles, syringes, and filters used (and admixture schedule card if utilized) should be placed back on the setup tray to be checked by a pharmacist. If the pharmacist approves the admixture, he or she initials the label next to the initials of the technician (figure 12.7).

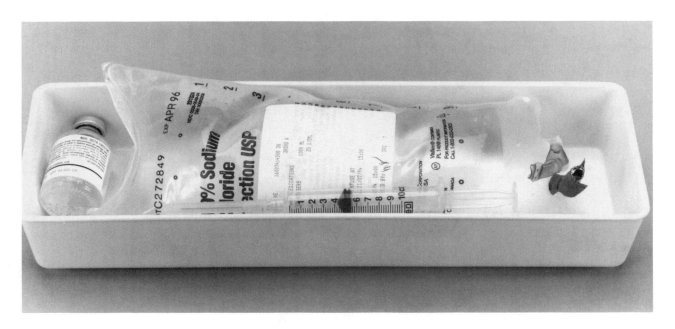

FIGURE 12.7. SETUP TRAY WITH COMPLETED ADMIXTURE

In noncomputerized programs, the schedule card, with the admixture order and any pretyped labels for the infusion series attached, should be filed alphabetically by patient or according to the next time the admixture is needed, depending on the procedures used in the pharmacy. This task is eliminated in a computerized system because the information is stored in the computer and can be recalled on the computer screen as needed.

STEP 10—TECHNICIAN DELIVERS ADMIXTURE TO PATIENT CARE AREA

The checked I.V. admixtures are then delivered to the proper patient care area. When admixtures are delivered, they should be placed inside a refrigerator specifically designated for them unless they are to be used immediately. Storing admixtures in a refrigerator prolongs their stability and provides a single location for a nurse to find an admixture for administration. The pharmacy technician should regularly check the supply of all admixtures already on that unit, noting the expiration date of each. Any outdated or discontinued admixtures should be returned to the pharmacy for credit and/or disposal.

STEPS 11, 12, 13—NURSE OBTAINS, VERIFIES, AND ADMINISTERS THE ADMIXTURE

The nurse obtains the admixture from the refrigerator just prior to the scheduled administration time; performs the final check on the admixture by comparing the label to a copy of the medication administration record; verifies that the patient name is correct; and then administers the admixture according to the physician's order and information known about the specific drug.

Nurses or physicians can telephone "stat" orders to the pharmacist when an I.V. admixture is needed immediately. The same steps are followed to process a stat order as those just described for routine admixtures. Before releasing the admixture, however, the pharmacist should check the prepared admixture for accuracy against the physician's written order sent to the pharmacy while the admixture was being prepared.

CHAPTER 13

QUALITY ASSURANCE AND PERFORMANCE IMPROVEMENT

QUALITY ASSURANCE FOR PHARMACY I.V. ADMIXTURE PROGRAMS

Quality assurance is a process to ensure that products and services meet standards of quality as defined by the organization and its customers. The American Society of Health-System Pharmacists has published a document, *ASHP Technical Assistance Bulletin on Quality Assurance for Pharmacy-Prepared Sterile Products* (Am J Hosp Pharm 1993; 50:2386-98), that is the most comprehensive reference available on quality assurance for pharmacy I.V. admixture programs. This document should be consulted for a complete discussion of this topic.

The ASHP technical assistance bulletin introduces the concept of risk level classification. Products are classified into one of three risk levels (risk level 1 being the lowest) based on risks to product integrity or patient safety. Most of the products prepared in pharmacy I.V. admixture programs are risk level 1 products, with very few being at risk level 3. This training manual has concentrated on techniques and procedures associated primarily with risk level 1. The risk level classification system is cumulative in that requirements for risk level 2 build on and are in addition to the requirements for risk level 1; risk level 3 requirements are in addition to risk level 2 requirements.

The three risk levels for preparing sterile products are based on such factors as how the products are stored and for how long; whether the products are prepared for one patient or are batch-prepared; whether the component products are initially sterile or nonsterile; and whether the products are prepared using a closed system or an open system.

Risk Level 1 This category includes products with the following characteristics:

- Storage time, including administration time, less than 28 hours at room temperature; less than 7 days under refrigeration; *OR* less than 30 days if frozen

- Sterile products without preservatives for individual patients; *OR* batch-prepared products with preservatives for multiple patients

- Sterile products transferred to sterile final containers (e.g., syringes, minibag)

Risk Level 2 This category includes products with the following characteristics:

- Storage time, including administration time, more than 28 hours at room temperature; more than 7 days under refrigeration; *OR* more than 30 days if frozen

- Batch-prepared products without preservatives for multiple patients

- Multiple sterile ingredients combined in a sterile reservoir by a closed-system aseptic transfer, then subdivided into multiple units

Risk Level 3 This category includes products with the following characteristics:

- Products compounded with nonsterile ingredients, containers, or equipment

- Sterile or nonsterile ingredients prepared in an open system, then terminally sterilized

The ASHP bulletin summarizes quality assurance standards in 11 different categories within each of the three risk levels to help pharmacists select the most appropriate procedures to follow. Those 11 categories within each risk level are:

- Policies and procedures
- Personnel education, training, and evaluation
- Storage and handling
- Facilities and equipment
- Garb
- Aseptic technique and product preparation
- Product validation
- Expiration dating
- Labeling
- End-product evaluation
- Documentation

The bulletin is a valuable source of practice standards in identifying problems or performance improvement opportunities in an I.V. admixture service.

PROCESS VALIDATION

In addition to a good training program in proper aseptic technique, pharmacists must develop other quality assurance programs. One of the best ways to monitor the quality of sterile compounding is through the use of process validation, which is sometimes referred to as process simulation or media fills. Process validation has been used historically by the pharmaceutical industry to ensure the sterility of manufactured products.

Process validation is a systematic test of the compounding process to ensure that personnel can demonstrate aseptic technique and that compounding processes produce sterile products. For most I.V. admixture operations, this involves simulating compounding procedures, using growth-promoting media (i.e., soybean broth) in place of the actual drug product.

Media fill validation is carried out using the same procedures and techniques used to prepare sterile products. The media fills are simply substituted for the normal drug and solution products. A number of routine aseptic manipulations that simulate the admixture process are made to the growth media to create a media fill unit, which is then incubated. Growth or cloudiness in the unit indicates microbial contamination, from either poor aseptic technique or a suboptimal compounding environment. An example of a commercially available validation test media kit is shown in figure 13.1.

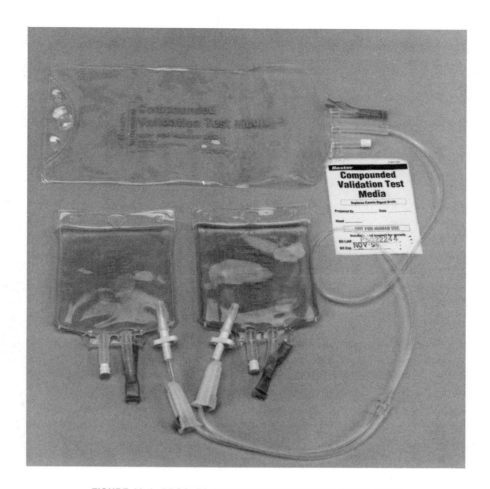

FIGURE 13.1. PROCESS VALIDATION TEST USING MEDIA FILLS

Media fill procedures can be used to simulate a variety of aseptic transfers, including syringes, transfer sets, and automated compounding devices. The number of media fill units prepared and aseptic manipulations made to each unit should reflect the most complex manipulations encountered in typical compounding situations. Therefore, the test would be more likely to show that personnel are capable of using effective aseptic technique to compound sterile products under fairly rigorous conditions. In addition to procedures and personnel, media fills can be used to validate a compounding facility.

A somewhat different approach to process validation is the use of solutions containing a fluorescein dye. This is particularly useful in evaluating aseptic technique associated with the preparation of chemotherapy agents because of the need to protect the operator, the environment, and the sterility of the drug. The actual process of compounding a sterile product is simulated with the use of dye-containing solutions substituted for actual drug product. Any aerosol droplets or spills can be seen readily when an ultraviolet light is shone into the work area, causing the fluorescein dye to glow. Thus, any "drug product" (i.e., simulated chemotherapy drug) outside the final solution container or the source vial is readily detected. Figure 13.2 illustrates this type of product.

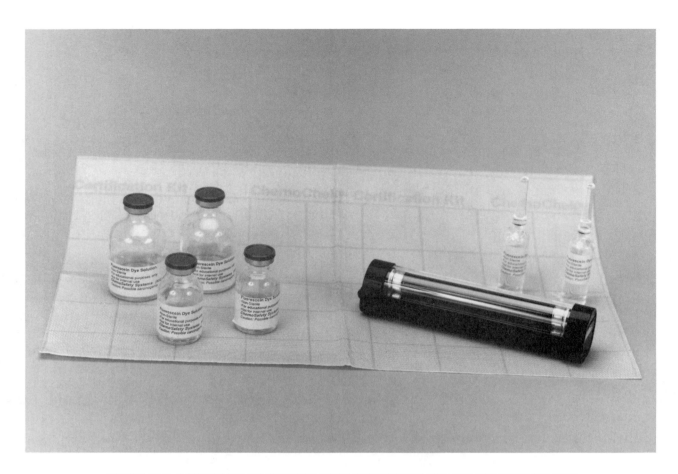

FIGURE 13.2. PROCESS VALIDATION TEST USING FLUORESCEIN DYE AND ULTRAVIOLET LIGHT

PERFORMANCE IMPROVEMENT

The past several years have seen tremendous growth in programs and information focused on quality. Many businesses have instituted quality or performance improvement programs under a variety of names such as total quality management, continuous quality improvement, and quality performance improvement in an effort to improve those processes critical to their products or services. The focus of the Joint Commission on Accreditation of Healthcare Organizations has evolved from the concept of quality assurance to continuous quality improvement and now emphasizes performance improvement. The term *performance improvement* will be used here because it is used by health systems accreditation agencies.

Regardless of the terminology used, these programs help guarantee that "right things are done right," i.e., pharmacy services are focused on the important aspects of patient needs and are provided in a high-quality, consistent manner. They also allow a pharmacy department to keep pace with changing situations by continuously focusing on ways to make things better. Performance improvement can be described as an ongoing systematic process for identifying improvement opportunities, developing solutions, and monitoring their effectiveness.

Steps in the Performance Improvement Process Although there are variations from one program to another, a performance improvement process typically consists of the following steps:

1. *Identify problems or improvement opportunities.* One way to identify improvement opportunities is to talk with the users of the pharmacy's products and services, i.e., the "customers," which include patients, nurses, physicians, pharmacy staff, suppliers, and others. A second way is to keep current on professional practice standards, accreditation standards, and legal and regulatory requirements. A third way is to seek out new ideas from articles in the pharmacy literature, visit other health care organizations, and attend professional pharmacy association meetings.

2. *Identify key individuals.* Once a process has been identified for improvement, the stakeholders should be determined and brought together. Stakeholders include individuals who provide the service or product, those who use the service or product, those who have responsibility for the process, and those who have influence or authority over the process.

3. *Analyze the situation.* The key individuals should establish a standard to be achieved, identify the current level of performance, and determine the gap that needs to be closed. The current process should be analyzed to understand how things actually work, identify problems or bottlenecks, and identify possible causes of the problems. Barriers and aids to closing the gap also need to be identified. During this step, it is important to focus on assuring that the new process can meet the needs of patients and other customers.

4. *Develop and implement solutions.* Several alternative solutions should be generated and evaluated. The solution selected may represent fine-tuning of the current process or developing an entirely new approach. It is important to keep in mind that nothing changes until the new or revised process is actually implemented. The focus at this point should be on action and results.

5. *Monitor results.* This is the feedback loop of the process to assure that the plan was successfully implemented and the results that were expected to be achieved actually were achieved. Information regarding the results of the performance improvement effort should be shared with appropriate staff and others.

Characteristics of Performance Improvement Programs High-quality performance programs have several characteristics in common:

1. The process is focused on meeting patient/customer needs.
2. Problem solving is done by teams.
3. Emphasis is on preventing errors.
4. Costs are actually lowered when quality is emphasized.
5. Emphasis is on correcting system errors.
6. Quality is everyone's responsibility.
7. Leadership supports innovation and calculated risk taking.
8. Quality issues drive decision making.
9. Quality is continuously measured and monitored.

High-quality products and services in an I.V. admixture program are moving targets. New drugs, supplies, technology, economic constraints, practice standards, and regulations are introduced on a continuous basis. To be satisfied with the status quo and not keep pace with a changing practice is to fall behind. Performance improvement programs go beyond allowing pharmacy personnel to react appropriately to change; they allow them the opportunity to be proactive in creating change.

APPENDIX A
SELECTED REFERENCES

Abramowitz PW, Hunt ML Jr. Principles and advantages of automated compounding: A pharmacy education guide. Deerfield, IL: Clintec Nutrition Co., 1992.

Achusim LE et al. Comparison of automated and manual methods of syringe filling. Am J Hosp Pharm 1990; 47:2492-5.

American Society of Hospital Pharmacists. ASHP accreditation standard for pharmacy technician training programs. Am J Hosp Pharm 1993; 50:124-6.

American Society of Hospital Pharmacists. ASHP guidelines: Minimum standards for pharmacists in institutions. Am J Hosp Pharm 1985; 42:372-5.

American Society of Hospital Pharmacists. ASHP technical assistance bulletin on hospital drug distribution and control. Am J Hosp Pharm 1980; 37:1097-1103.

American Society of Hospital Pharmacists. ASHP technical assistance bulletin on handling cytotoxic and hazardous drugs. Am J Hosp Pharm 1990; 47:1033-49.

American Society of Hospital Pharmacists. ASHP technical assistance bulletin on outcome competencies and training guidelines for institutional pharmacy technician training programs. Am J Hosp Pharm 1982; 39:317-20.

American Society of Hospital Pharmacists. ASHP technical assistance bulletin on quality assurance for pharmacy-prepared sterile products. Am J Hosp Pharm 1993; 50:2386-98.

American Society of Hospital Pharmacists. Aseptic preparation of parenteral products (videotape and study guide). Bethesda, MD: the Society, 1985.

Anderson RW. Technicians and the future of pharmacy. Am J Hosp Pharm 1987; 44:1593-7.

Anon. Manual for pharmacy technicians. Bethesda, MD: American Society of Hospital Pharmacists, 1993.

Barker KN, ed. Recommendations of the NCCLVP for the compounding and administration of intravenous solutions. Bethesda, MD: American Society of Hospital Pharmacists, 1981.

Boylan JC. Essential elements of quality control. Am J Hosp Pharm 1983; 40:1936-9.

Brier KL. Evaluating aseptic technique of pharmacy personnel. Am J Hosp Pharm 1983; 40:400-3.

Bryan D, Marback RC. Laminar-airflow equipment certification: What the pharmacist needs to know. Am J Hosp Pharm 1984; 41:1343-9.

Centers for Disease Control. Guideline for handwashing and hospital environmental control. Am J Infect Control 1986; 4(8): 110-29.

Clark T et al. Quality assurance for pharmacy-prepared sterile products (videotape and workbook). Bethesda, MD: American Society of Hospital Pharmacists, 1994.

Cohen MR. Proper technique for handling parenteral products. Hosp Pharm 1986; 21:1106.

Crawford SY et al. National survey of quality assurance activities for pharmacy-prepared sterile products in hospitals. Am J Hosp Pharm 1991; 48:2398-2413.

Dirks I et al. Method for testing aseptic technique of intravenous admixture personnel. Am J Hosp Pharm 1982; 39:457-9.

Donnelly AJ, Djuric M. Cardioplegia solutions. Am J Hosp Pharm 1991; 48:2444-60.

Food and Drug Administration. Safety alert: Hazards of precipitation associated with parenteral nutrition. Am J Hosp Pharm. 1994; 51:1427-8.

Godwin HN, Shoup LK. Implementation guide: Centralized intravenous admixture program. Deerfield, IL: Travenol Laboratories, 1977.

Hanold LS et al. Implementation of a self-directed pharmacy technician training program. Am J Hosp Pharm 1982; 39:446-9.

Hasegawa GR, ed. Caring about stability and compatibility. Am J Hosp Pharm 1994; 51:1533-4.

Hunt ML Jr. Intravenous admixture training program for pharmacy personnel. Am J Hosp Pharm 1974; 31:467-71.

Kalman MK et al. Increasing pharmacy productivity by expanding the role of pharmacy technicians. Am J Hosp Pharm 1992; 49:84-9.

King JC. Guide to parenteral admixtures. St. Louis: Kabi Vitrum, 1994

Kirschenbaum BE, Latiolais CJ. Injectable medications: A guide to stability and reconstitution. New York: Organon Inc., 1994.

Leff RD, Roberts RJ. Practical aspects of intravenous drug administration, 2nd ed. Bethesda, MD: American Society of Hospital Pharmacists, 1992.

Lindly CM, Deloatch KH. Infusion technology manual and videotape: A self-instructional approach. Bethesda, MD: American Society of Hospital Pharmacists, 1993.

Mirtallo JM. The complexity of mixing calcium and phosphate. Am J Hosp Pharm 1994; 51:1535-6.

McDiarmid MA. Medical surveillance for antineoplastic-drug handlers. Am J Hosp Pharm 1990; 47:1061-6.

McKinnon BT, Avis KE. Membrane filtration of pharmaceutical solutions. Am J Hosp Pharm 1993; 50:1921-36.

Morris BG et al. Quality-control plan for intravenous admixture programs. II: Validation of operator technique. Am J Hosp Pharm 1980; 37:668-72.

National Coordinating Committee on Large Volume Parenterals. Recommended methods for compounding intravenous admixtures in Hospitals. Am J Hosp Pharm 1975; 32:261-70.

National Coordinating Committee on Large Volume Parenterals. Recommended guidelines for quality assurance in hospital centralized intravenous admixture services. Am J Hosp Pharm 1980; 37:645-55.

National Coordinating Committee on Large Volume Parenterals. Recommendations for the labeling of large volume parenterals. Am J Hosp Pharm 1978; 35:49-51.

National Coordinating Committee on Large Volume Parenterals. Recommended standard of practice, policies, and procedures for intravenous therapy. Am J Hosp Pharm 1980; 37:660-3.

National Coordinating Committee on Large Volume Parenterals. Recommended procedure for in-use testing of large volume parenterals suspected of contamination or of producing a reaction in a patient. Am J Hosp Pharm 1978; 35:678-82.

National Coordinating Committee on Large Volume Parenterals. Recommended system for surveillance and reporting of problems with large volume parenterals in hospitals. Am J Hosp Pharm 1975; 34:1251-3.

Peters BG et al. Certification program in antineoplastic drug preparation for pharmacy technicians and pharmacists. Am J Hosp Pharm 1994; 51:1902-6.

Phelps SJ, Cochran EB, eds. Guidelines for administration of intravenous medications to pediatric patients. Bethesda, MD: American Society of Hospital Pharmacists, 1993.

Phillips DJM, Smith JE. Six-month hospital pharmacy-based technician training program. Am J Hosp Pharm 1984; 41:2614-8.

Power LA et al. Update on safe handling of hazardous drugs: The advice of experts. Am J Hosp Pharm 1990; 47:1050-60.

Ray MD, ed. Training hospital pharmacy technicians. Am J Hosp Pharm 1984; 41:2595-6.

Rich DS. Evaluation of a disposable, elastomeric infusion device in the home environment. Am J Hosp Pharm 1992; 49:1712-6.

Sebastian G, Thielke TS. Work analysis of an admixture service. Am J Hosp Pharm 1983; 40:2149-53.

Scope of Pharmacy Practice Project. Summary of the final report of the Scope of Pharmacy Practice Project. Am J Hosp Pharm 1994; 2179-82.

Strozyk WR, Underwood DA. Development and benefits of a pharmacy technician career ladder. Am J Hosp Pharm 1994; 51:666-9.

Trissel LA, ed. Compounding our problems. Am J Hosp Pharm 1994; 51:1534.

Trissel LA. Handbook on injectable drugs, 8th ed. Bethesda, MD: American Society of Hospital Pharmacists, 1994.

Turco S, King RE. Extemporaneous preparation. In: Turco S, King RE, eds. Sterile dosage forms. Philadelphia: Lea & Febiger, 1987:55-61.

Vaida AJ, Gabos C. Intravenous admixture systems. In: Brown TR, ed. Handbook of institutional pharmacy practice. Bethesda, MD: American Society of Hospital Pharmacists, 1992; 175-92.

APPENDIX B
TRADE NAMES AND COPYRIGHT OWNERS

Presented here is a list of trade names mentioned in this manual, along with the owners of the trademarks or registered trademarks. With some exceptions, as in lists such as this one and the list of pharmaceuticals in chapter 3, trade names may be accompanied by the symbols ™ (trademark) or ® (registered trademark) to indicate that use of the name is restricted to the trademark owner. The informal symbol ™ often is used with unregistered marks to indicate a claim of common law trademark rights. Once a trademark application has been filed, examined, and approved and the certificate of trademark registration has been received, the symbol ® may be used with the applicable trademark, followed by the generic name.

Trade Name	Owner of Trademark or Registered Trademark
ADD-Vantage	Abbott Laboratories
Alferon N	Purdue Frederick Company
Amikin	Apothecon
Ancef	SmithKline Beecham Pharmaceuticals
Atgam	The Upjohn Company
Automix Automated Compounder	Clintec Nutrition Co.
Azactam	Bristol-Myers Squibb Co.
Bactrim	Roche Laboratories
Baxa pump	Baxa Corp.
BiCNU	Bristol-Myers Squibb Oncology Division
Blenoxane	Bristol-Myers Squibb Oncology Division
CeeNU	Bristol-Myers Squibb Oncology Division
Cerubidine	Wyeth-Ayerst Laboratories
Cefobid	Roerig Division (Pfizer Inc.)
Cefotan	Stuart Pharmaceuticals
Cefizox	Fujisawa USA
Cipro	Miles, Pharmaceutical Division
Claforan	Hoechst-Roussel Pharmaceuticals
Cleocin	The Upjohn Company
Cosmegen	Merck & Co.
Cytosar-U	The Upjohn Company
Cytovene	Syntex Laboratories
Cytoxan	Bristol-Myers Squibb Oncology Division
Decadron	Merck & Co.
Diflucan	Roerig Division (Pfizer Inc.)
Dobutrex	Eli Lilly and Company
Flagyl	SCS Pharmaceuticals
Flashball	Baxter International Inc.
Floxin	McNeil Pharmaceutical Corp.
Fortaz	Glaxo Pharmaceuticals
Foscavir	Astra USA
Fungizone	Apothecon
Gammagard	Baxter International Inc.
Gammar	Armour Pharmaceutical Co.
Gamimune N	Miles, Pharmaceutical Division Biological Products

Garamycin	Schering Corp.
HepatAmine	McGaw Inc.
Hexadrol	Organon
Humulin	Eli Lilly and Company
Hydrocortone	Merck & Co.
Idamycin	Pharmacia Adria
IFEX	Bristol-Myers Squibb Oncology Division
Imuran	Burroughs Wellcome
Intron A	Schering Corp.
Intropin	Du Pont Pharma
Isuprel	Sanofi Winthrop Pharmaceuticals
Kefzol	Eli Lilly and Company
Kefurox	Eli Lilly and Company
Kytril	SmithKline Beecham Pharmaceuticals
Leukine	Immunex Corp.
Luer-Lok	Beckton Dickinson & Co.
Lupron	TAP Pharmaceuticals
Mefoxin	Merck & Co.
Mezlin	Miles, Pharmaceutical Division
Micromedex	Micromedex
Micromix Compounder	Clintec Nutrition Co.
Mini-Bag Plus Container	Baxter International Inc.
Minocin	Lederle Laboratories
Mithracin	Miles, Pharmaceutical Division
Monistat	Janssen Pharmaceutica
Monocid	SmithKline Beecham Pharmaceuticals
Mutamycin	Bristol-Myers Squibb Oncology Division
Nebcin	Eli Lilly and Company
Neosar	Pharmacia Adria
Neupogen	Amgen Inc.
Nipent	Parke-Davis
Nipride	Roche Laboratories
Novantrone	Lederle Laboratories
Novolin	Novo Nordisk Pharmaceuticals
Omnipen-N	Wyeth-Ayerst Laboratories
Oncovin	Eli Lilly and Company
Orthoclone OKT3	Ortho Biotech
Paraplatin	Bristol-Myers Squibb Oncology Division
Pentam	Fujisawa USA
Pepcid	Merck & Co.
Pfizerpen	Roerig Division (Pfizer Inc.)
Pharm-Aide Fluid Dispensing System	Baxter International Inc.
Pipracil	Lederle Laboratories
Pitocin	Parke-Davis
Platinol	Bristol-Myers Squibb Oncology Division
Polygam	American Red Cross
Primaxin	Merck & Co.
Prokine	Hoechst-Roussel Pharmaceuticals
Proleukin	Chiron Therapeutics
RenAmin	Clintec Nutrition Co.
Retrovir	Burroughs Wellcome
Rocephin	Roche Laboratories

Roferon-A	Roche Laboratories
Sandimmune	Sandoz Pharmaceuticals Corp.
Sandoglobulin	Sandoz Pharmaceuticals Corp.
Sandostatin	Sandoz Pharmaceuticals Corp.
Septra	Burroughs Wellcome
Solu-Cortef	The Upjohn Company
Solu-Medrol	The Upjohn Company
Tagamet	SmithKline Beecham Pharmaceuticals
Tazicef	SmithKline Beecham Pharmaceuticals
Tazidime	Eli Lilly and Company
Timentin	SmithKline Beecham Pharmaceuticals
Travasol	Clintec Nutrition Co.
Tridil	Du Pont Pharma
Unasyn	Roerig Division (Pfizer Inc.)
Unipen	Wyeth-Ayerst Laboratories
Vancocin	Eli Lilly and Company
Vancoled	Lederle Standard Products
Velban	Eli Lilly and Company
VePesid	Bristol-Myers Squibb Oncology Division
Viaflex Plus Container	Baxter International Inc.
Vibramycin	Roerig Division (Pfizer Inc.)
Vira-A	Parke-Davis
Xylocaine	Astra USA
Zanosar	The Upjohn Company
Zantac	Glaxo Pharmaceuticals
Zefazone	The Upjohn Company
Zinacef	Glaxo Pharmaceuticals
Zofran	Cerenex
Zosyn	Lederle Laboratories
Zovirax	Burroughs Wellcome

Date Due

ILL (YMM)		
720 6824		
OCT 2 4 1997		
ILL (HBP)		
9778824		
FEB 2 0 1998		
ILL (BRB)		
6x4 850		
MAY 2 7 1999		
ILL (NJQ)		
1733529		
OCT 0 1 2000		

PRINTED IN U.S.A.   CAT. NO. 24 161